G000280598

Let's talk

Let's talk...

about
relationships,
sex and intimacy

Richie Sadlier

Gill Books

Gill Books
Hume Avenue
Park West
Dublin 12
www.gillbooks.ie

Gill Books is an imprint of M.H. Gill and Co.

9780717191901

Designed by Bartek Janczak
Illustrations on page 74–76 by Derry Dillon
Edited by Esther Ní Dhonnacha
Printed by CPI Group (UK) Ltd, Croydon, CRO 4YY
This book is typeset in 10.5 on 16.5pt Calluna.

*The paper used in this book comes from the wood pulp of
sustainably managed forests.*

A CIP catalogue record for this book is available from the
British Library.

5 4 3 2 1

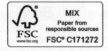

For my fifteen-year-old self

Contents

Introduction

Let's talk ... about sex and relationships. Let's talk about dating, sexting, drinking and break-ups and all the things you might be learning from porn. Let's talk about pleasure and fun, condoms and safety, and all the ways to understand consent. **Let's talk about the stuff *you* want to talk about.** The stuff *you* really want to learn. The stuff *you* want to understand. Let's talk about being single, being a boyfriend, being gay and being straight. Let's talk about it all.

Let's not do what previous generations of Irish people did. Let's actually talk about this stuff so that when the time comes for you to make certain decisions or have certain experiences, you'll be better informed and prepared for things to go well. You won't get everything right – nor will your partners, for that matter – but you'll have a far better chance of positive experiences if you've had the chance to talk, read and learn about these things in advance.

HOW THIS BOOK CAME ABOUT

I wish I was handed a book like this when I was in my mid-teens. Back then, people didn't spend much time talking to young people about sex and relationships. Like every generation before us, we were left to learn for ourselves, mainly from our own mistakes. Teachers didn't go into much detail about anything, and parents were unsure of how much to say. On top of that, most of us were probably too shy or awkward to ask certain questions. I'm not sure why exactly, but it was considered wrong or perverted if you showed too much of an interest in anything to do with sex, especially as a teenage boy, so we rarely brought up the topic with adults. As a result, we all headed into adulthood without any meaningful or helpful sex education. As you can imagine, this was an approach that didn't work out well for everyone. Looking back, I can definitely say it didn't work out well for me.

The truth is, a book like this could never have been published in Ireland when I was your age. It wasn't acceptable back then to give young people the kind of information that's in these chapters. However, the more insight I get into the lives of teenagers in Ireland today, the more I think it would be *un*acceptable if something like this wasn't available for you to read. If you've been given this book by an adult in your life, they must think you're emotionally intelligent and mature enough to understand this content. Or, to put it another way, they think you're ready.

So how did this book come about? First of all, if you've watched any Republic of Ireland or Champions League matches on RTÉ over the past decade, you probably know I work as a football pundit. My role is to analyse the games and the performance of everyone involved, and give my opinions on what's going well and what needs to improve. Whether you already knew this or you're just finding it out now, I want you to know that job has nothing to do with me writing this book.

Away from the television cameras, I do work of a very different kind. I'm an adolescent psychotherapist, and the majority of my clients are teenage lads. This job gives me the chance to help young people, but it also gives me the opportunity to understand their lives. I hear them speak about their worries and concerns, their hopes and ambitions. They explain the challenges they have and the opportunities they want. They talk about the realities of their lives as teenagers today and all the things that are important to them. In other words, they talk honestly about what it's like to be them in the world today, and they come to therapy looking for guidance and support.

The more openly young people spoke to me, particularly about sex and sexuality, the more it was clear they needed direction and support. In 2016, I co-created a module in sexual health for Transition Year students in an all-boys school. The more time I spent in the classroom, the more I understood the students' hunger for information and the right advice. I was invited to talk in different schools and sports clubs about this topic. Every time I spoke about this stuff, it became more obvious how much it was appreciated by the young people listening. I spoke on podcasts, television programmes and radio shows about the need to support young people's development in this area, and every time I did, parents would contact me saying they needed help too.

It's clear how much things have changed in this area compared to when I was a teenager. It seems people in this country are ready and willing to embrace new ways of supporting you and your friends to learn about the richness and variety of relationships and sexuality. **It's totally normal for you to want to learn about sex, after all; we adults just needed time to realise we needed a new approach to helping you out.**

A book about these topics could be useful to any young person, but I've decided to focus on the experiences of young men in this area. Writing a book that focuses on teenage lads isn't a statement of neglect or disinterest in everyone else. It's a response to a particular need that I've observed from countless hours working to support teenage lads in my therapy practice and in schools.

HOW TO USE THIS BOOK

If you were given the job of devising the sex education curriculum for your school, what would you include? Where would you start if you had to decide what every teenager your age should be taught? It's a tricky question, isn't it?

Don't be too bothered if you feel a little bamboozled by a task like this, because it's far from straightforward. Adults have never agreed on this. If I asked a hundred people the same question, I'd probably get a hundred different answers. It would be impossible to get everyone to sign off on the one approach, that's for sure. Everyone has their own attitude to sex and their own view of what young people should be taught. Some people think less is more when it comes to sex education, meaning young people should be left to pick up most of their education from real-life experiences. Others think it should depend entirely on the religious beliefs of the parents, or the ethical approach of the school they happen to attend. One thing's for sure: this isn't a topic people will ever agree on.

Now, if I asked you what should be included in a book like this, what would you say? In other words, what information do lads your age really want about sex? What guidance do you think you need when it comes to relationships? Maybe you already think you know enough from everything you've seen in porn, but can you think of any lessons you need to learn that porn doesn't teach?

Books about sex and relationships can be written in many different ways, but the approach here is to be open, frank, informative, personal and honest. You might find certain chapters more interesting than others. You will certainly be drawn to some topics more than others. It's possible some of the issues and questions seem irrelevant in your life now, but remember they may well be important for you some time in the future.

Every chapter will include a brief explanation about how we avoided speaking about these topics in the past. 'Let's not talk' will be a quick look back at how this approach prevented teenagers getting the kind of information and guidance that could have been really useful. I've included this because I think you'll understand the potential benefits of talking more openly about this stuff the more you learn how damaging it was in the past to stay quiet about it.

And just so you know, being able to talk about sex and relationships doesn't mean you have to have all the answers. Actually, sometimes it's just about knowing which questions to ask and when to listen. It really doesn't mean you have to know everything. It certainly doesn't mean you get to tell other people what they should and shouldn't do in their personal lives. It just means you've reached the stage where you know the benefits of seeking advice or asking for guidance. It means you realise how helpful it is to talk openly to someone you trust and that you have the confidence and the vocabulary to say what you mean. On top of that, it means you know the downsides of trying to solve every issue you face on your own. It means you understand that we all have different experiences and opinions in this area. The more we share them with one another the more we'll all learn.

Each chapter will have a very brief account of some of my memories or experiences with each topic from my teenage years. I figured it would be a bit hypocritical if I kept saying how healthy it is to talk openly about these topics if I wasn't going to say anything personal myself to kick things off.

I'll share details of many of the discussions and debates that took place in the sexual health workshops I delivered to teenagers in schools and sports clubs. I'll describe some of the situations that clients of mine have faced in their own lives. 'Lessons from the Therapy Room' will give you an insight into the real-life scenarios that people have faced and some of the things that could be learned from how they behaved. Obviously, I've changed all of their names and some other details to make sure it's impossible for anyone to identify them.

We'll be covering the topic of sexual orientation and some of the issues that can come up for people in this area. (Spoiler: it's completely fine if you are still unsure about this or if you're still questioning your own orientation.) We'll explore the world of relationships and some of the challenges and dilemmas that can arise between partners. It wouldn't be possible to mention all the reasons that relationships come to an end, but we'll cover the importance and benefits of breaking up in a healthy way.

We'll also venture deep into the world of pornography, looking at the role it can play in young people's sex education. I'll describe the many ways you and your partners can protect yourselves from unplanned or unwanted consequences of sexual activity. There's also a chapter on consent, which will add to your understanding of why it is so important. We'll finish by looking at how alcohol can impact people's thoughts and behaviours in all of these areas.

ADOLESCENT SEXUALITY

You're too old at this stage for me to bang on about the bodily changes that occur during puberty. I'm sure you'd just feel patronised if I started to explain it to you now. I assume someone covered that with you when you were approaching the end of primary school, but you've moved on now to a higher level of understanding of yourself and your body. You're ready now to start learning more about your emerging sexuality, and about the ways it can impact you and your behaviour.

By now, I'm pretty sure you know what it's like to feel aroused. It's usually not something people talk about comfortably and openly with one another, but it's an entirely healthy occurrence for lads your age. In other words, it's perfectly normal to regularly get an erection if you're an adolescent male, even if it sometimes happens at the least convenient times! **Whether in class, on the bus, watching TV or walking your dog, there is always a possibility something will set you off**. (I have no doubt you are already aware of this!)

Many lads feel uncomfortable getting an unexpected erection. They feel as if there's something wrong with them, or that maybe they're more excitable than they should be. It's certainly not something they're happy to chat about over dinner with siblings and parents. So given it's something that's probably rarely spoken about, it's worth giving a brief explanation of the impact it can have.

First of all, an erection can happen at any time of the day or night. It can even happen while you're asleep. It can be triggered by any number of things to begin with. You might see something or hear something. Maybe you remembered something or imagined something. Once this happens, the body takes over. Your brain releases nitric oxide, which dilates blood vessels, and blood then rushes to your penis as quickly as possible, causing you to experience an erection. You might not welcome it if this happens while you're surrounded by other people, but it's a natural bodily response to feeling aroused in the first place.

That's the physical part explained, but there's an equally important psychological impact too. This may also be something you're already familiar with, but an erection isn't just a bodily sensation. It comes with an urge to act! The power of arousal can be pretty overwhelming at times, particularly during adolescence, which often leads to behaviour which is impulsive and 'in the moment'.

I'll put it this way: if an erection could communicate, it would have no interest whatsoever in discussing the long-term consequences of sexual behaviour. It would laugh you out of the room if you suggested taking things slowly. It would be screaming at you to act now! In fact, it would probably be disappointed in you if you tried to talk it down in favour of sensibly considering the alternatives to sexual activity. So, given the influence it can have over you and your behaviour, it's important to learn ways of handling a situation when you have one.

Before I go on, I don't want you thinking I'm giving erections a hard time here (pardon the pun!). As I said already, it's perfectly normal for sexually healthy lads to experience this. However, extra focus is needed in those few moments when you consider your options before you act. In other words, the 'thinking time' between feeling the initial impulse and the moment you act. Obviously, many people have wonderful experiences by acting entirely on impulse, but it's an approach that can have pretty negative outcomes too. This certainly applies to scenarios involving sexual arousal.

It's not OK to lose all control of your behaviour because you're aroused. It's a cop-out to say you had no choices. One of the aims of this book is to help you figure out the 'thinking time' for yourself. To help you to be able to make sound decisions. To help you make the most out of any situation you face. To help you maximise the amount of fun you have while limiting the difficulty you cause for yourself or others. Basically, this book is here to help you think about how you'd like to be as a sexual person and to learn how to enjoy this area of your life as much as possible.

IT'S TIME TO TALK

It might not feel like it sometimes, but you have more freedom now than you've ever had. You've come a long way from the days when you had to hold someone else's hand to cross a road. You can now own your own phone, you can go on the internet alone and you're approaching the stage when you can start to earn your own money. There was a time when you would never have been left unsupervised, when you couldn't go anywhere on your own and at least one of your parents knew who you were with at all times. You were considered too young to be trusted to make decisions for yourself, so the adults in your life constantly made them for you. No matter how you felt about it, you were under the watchful eye of others all the time. That's the way life is for most people during childhood.

IT'S VERY
NORMAL TO
WANT MORE
FREEDOM,
SPACE AND
PRIVACY
THE OLDER
YOU GET.

In just a few years' time, your situation is going to be very different. You'll have reached adulthood and there will be very few limits on the kind of choices you can make. If you can afford the flight, you can travel to the other side of the world if you want. You can live where you want, hang out with whoever you like, and spend your free time doing anything you choose.

Your parents may still want to stay informed and know a lot about your life, but there will be huge chunks of information you deliberately hold back from them. That's the way things are meant to be by the time you're an adult. Moving from your childhood levels of privacy (i.e. none!) to adulthood levels of privacy (i.e. loads!) can be a bumpy journey for many young people and their parents, but it's very normal to want more freedom, space and privacy the older you get.

One of the many tricky aspects of this journey is knowing which parts to keep private and which issues to discuss. On the one hand, you may want to have experiences that are personal to you, or private between you and your partners. But you mightn't always have the knowledge or experience that could really help. You mightn't be comfortable seeking information, guidance or advice, but you also realise there's a lot you don't yet know. This is certainly the case for most teenagers when it comes to their sexuality.

I know it can often be awkward to speak about really personal things. And it can be difficult to know how to start certain conversations. **By staying quiet about what you're going through,**

however, you may end up cutting yourself off from getting information and advice that would really help. The thing is, while you have a right to privacy in this area of your life, and you might prefer to keep several elements of your personal life to yourself, it's not necessarily a healthy thing to keep quiet about *everything* you're going through.

Sometimes an online search will help you to find the information you need, but there are loads of scenarios where Google won't be able to help. In many cases, a conversation with someone you trust will be required. There are times when it's sensible to ask a mate for their opinion on something, but other times the best person to talk to is your partner. In some scenarios, it's wise to ask a guidance counsellor for advice, or to speak in confidence about an issue with a GP. And even though you might not feel like it, there are times when a parent is the right person to approach.

Like everyone else, you will find a way that works for you over time on a trial-and-error basis. In the meantime, as your curiosity and interest in sex are developing, I hope this book can provide you with guidance that you find useful. I hope it helps you grow your understanding of many of the issues that come up for people in this area of their lives. I hope it enhances your awareness of matters that will be important for you soon and helps you tease out for yourself what kind of relationships would work for you. I want it to help you realise the benefits of talking openly about sex and sexuality while also grasping the importance of guarding your own privacy. Basically, I want you to think smartly and be clued in when it comes to sex.

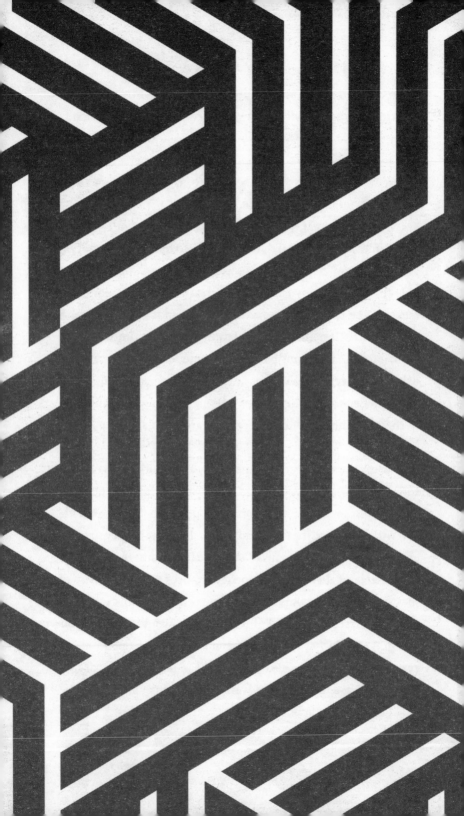

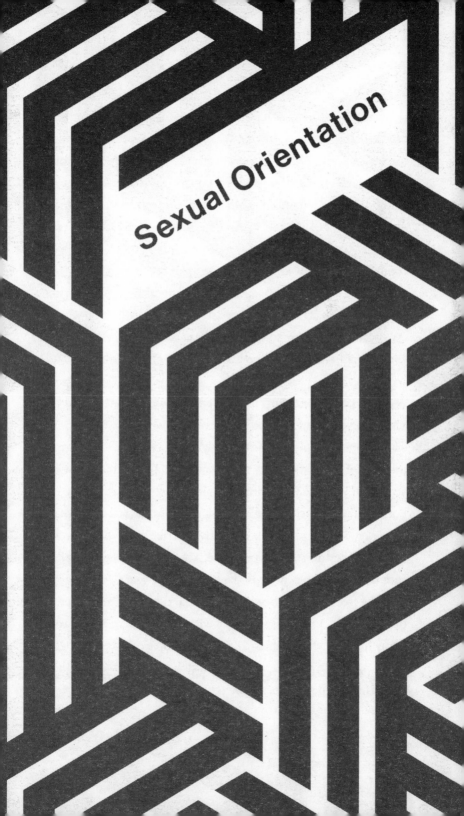

Sexual Orientation

Think back to the last time you felt sexually aroused. Can you remember what sparked it off? For example, was it something you saw or something you heard? Was it caused by something that was said to you, maybe? Or was it a thought that came into your head? Maybe it was the result of something you read or something you remembered? It could have been a mix of these things, obviously, or it could have been something entirely different too.

Your mind is probably racing through loads of different memories you have in this area (which is possibly affecting your ability to focus on reading this!) but let me ask you another question which is particularly relevant to what we'll be covering now: How would you describe the person who was the focus of your arousal?

Your sexual orientation is about who you are attracted to and who you want to have relationships with. The traditional way to approach this topic is to neatly file every man on the planet into one of four categories. You're gay if you like men and you're straight if you like women. You're bisexual if you're attracted to both and you're asexual if you find you're attracted to neither. However, while these labels perfectly describe many people's orientation, they don't fit for everyone. The list of ways to describe your orientation has increased a lot in recent years. People now have the freedom to go beyond traditional categories and descriptions to find a term they connect with. While there are far too many for me to name them all here, remember there is no right or wrong way to describe your orientation. All that counts is that the term you choose works for you.

For many people, this area is pretty straightforward. They know who they like and they don't have a problem with it. Maybe that's you? Others have no idea who they like and they don't have a problem with that either. That could be you too. There are plenty of lads, however, who are concerned about this aspect of themselves and are unsure where to go for support or reassurance. This chapter is about some of the questions and issues that arise for some of you reading this book who are either questioning your sexuality, or who know you're not straight. If that's you, then hopefully this section will be of some help.

Before you read on, this might be a good point for me to introduce the topic of gender. Firstly, because gender identity has become an increasingly important area for many young people, and secondly, because many people seem to confuse sexual orientation with gender identity. Just to explain the difference: your sexual orientation is about the people you are attracted to, while gender identity is all about who you *are*. Terms like *cisgender*, *transgender* and *nonbinary* are some of the labels that fit for people when they discuss their gender identity, but they're not forms of sexual orientation. Some people describe their sexual orientation in terms of the gender identity of their partners – so these two topics do overlap – but it's important to realise they're not the same. That's a whole other book, but for now ... back to the topic of this one! And while I want to acknowledge how important your gender identity may be to you, this section is about sexual orientation.

Me and sexual orientation

I knew I was attracted to girls from a young age. I didn't have a spell during my teenage years when I wondered about my sexual orientation, like many people do. Terms like *pansexual*, *bicurious* and *heteroflexible* just weren't in my world, so I didn't spend any time considering which label to go with. It sounds like I'm describing a much simpler time, but back then I thought people could identify only as gay, straight or bisexual. I don't recall any memories of questioning whether I wanted to be in relationships with lads, but I have several memories where it was pretty clear I liked girls. Not all memories from our early adolescence are ones we are happy for other people to know, something I'm sure you can relate to, but here's one I remember from when I was 11.

I was staying in London with relatives, and each day myself and my cousin headed off to the newsagent to buy football stickers (they were a big thing back then!). The daily trip was the high point of my time in London because it gave me the chance to open page 3 of *The Sun* newspaper to feast my little 11-year-old eyes on that day's picture of a topless woman (this was also a big thing to me back then!). Boobs weren't something I was able to see anywhere else – the internet didn't exist at the time – so I wasn't going to pass up the opportunity each morning to take a look. The reason I remember this so clearly is that on the third trip to the shop, the man behind the counter asked me to stop looking at something I wasn't going to buy and the three other people in the shop just stared at me and laughed. Obviously, I went bright red and got really embarrassed and I never went back to that shop again.

I could share countless other examples, but I'll save you the hassle of reading them all. I used to be embarrassed by sharing stories like this, but now I realise that it's perfectly healthy and normal to be curious and excited by nudity around that age. We all have our own journey when it comes to how our sexuality emerges, but it was always clear to me that I was heterosexual.

Let's *not* talk about sexual orientation

Sexual orientation wasn't openly discussed when I went to school. The only relationships that were considered healthy and normal were ones between men and women, so they were the only kind of relationship that we covered back then. There may have been some passing mentions of homosexuality in certain classes, but that was it. Just to illustrate how different things were back then, it was actually illegal for two men to have sex in Ireland when I first joined secondary school. (The law was changed and it was decriminalised the following year, in 1993.) It's pretty mad to think that a country would pass a law that bans a type of sexuality, but that's how it was back then (by the way, it's still that way today in over 60 countries!). So, if you were a teenager at the time who was questioning your sexuality, or you knew you weren't heterosexual, knowing where to go for information, support or guidance would have been tricky.

I didn't have any openly gay friends growing up, and I didn't know of any openly gay couples in my area. I know now that one of my best mates – my sister Anna – was gay all along. Some of the lads I played football with were gay, classmates were gay, and some of my parents' friends were gay. For their own personal reasons, they all made choices not to speak openly about it, and from what I remember about how things were back then, I wouldn't blame them.

Things have changed a lot since those days, but it can still be uncomfortable for young people to begin conversations about their own sexual orientation for fear of the reaction they'll get from other people. Shyness can get in the way too, but also, many lads just prefer to keep this area of their lives private from those around them until they are more comfortable opening up. **I've never known anyone who felt anxious about telling others they were heterosexual, but it can be very different for people who think they're not.** Many teenagers are still unsure where to go for information on this area, which is why I think it's important to cover it here.

QUESTIONING

When it comes to understanding our sexual orientation and real-ising what kinds of relationships and partners we want, not all of us find the answers at the same age. And just to complicate things a little further, not all of us stick to the first answer we come up with either.

YOUR SEXUAL
ORIENTATION
IS JUST AS
IMPORTANT
AND VALID
AS ANYONE
ELSE'S

For many people, there is no uncertainty or doubt. They have a clear idea where they stand on this issue. For others – maybe for you or some of your friends – this is a question that has still to be answered. Given that adolescence is all about working out who you are over time, it's entirely normal for this question to be an issue at your age. **You're at a stage of life where it's healthy to be working out who you are, but remember you're not expected to have all the answers straight away.** This is particularly the case for many people when it comes to their sexual orientation.

In fact, it's really important not to label yourself prematurely. For example, Paddy, a 16-year-old client of mine, was questioning his orientation (and his gender identity). He just described himself as being with whatever partner he was with at the time. 'Myself and Jay are together,' for example. This worked better for him than trying to categorise himself, his partners, his relationships, his gender or his orientation. When we discussed these issues in sessions, he said things like 'I'm with Jay at the moment, and I don't need to define things beyond that.' This was really effective because it gave him more time to explore these questions himself without expectations or pressure to come up with an answer.

You may already have a strong opinion about which description fits you best, or like many people your age, you may be unsure. In other words, you're either questioning your sexual orientation or you're not. And if you *are* questioning, I want you to know that it's perfectly normal and appropriate for you to be doing this at your age. Even though it's normal to still be trying to work out who you are, it can often be a distressing and confusing issue for many young people.

So, what are you supposed to do if you're questioning? Well, many people who are curious about this issue in their own lives find it helpful to explore different aspects of their sexuality. They may have gay experiences, for example. To some people, these experiences are just sexual exploration (in other words, trying different things), but to others, they can be important steps towards finding – and understanding – their sexual orientation. If you or someone you know is in this situation, the best advice is to avoid putting yourself under pressure to stick tightly to one label and don't put yourself under time pressure to answer this question once and for all. Just like Paddy did, try to stay flexible in your thinking and keep an open mind.

Also, if you are spending a lot of time stressing over how other people are going to react and what they'll think of you if you speak openly about this, you need to know that you won't always be this concerned with what others think. You know how you've sometimes felt really embarrassed or awkward in loads of situations over the last couple of years? Have you noticed you have become self-conscious about stuff now in ways you weren't when you were much younger? (Your body shape, your appearance, your popularity?) This is because you are at a stage of your life when you are most sensitive to what other people think of you. The bad news is that this is an unavoidable part of life for most lads your age, but the good news is that this doesn't last for much longer. It can sound really patronising to young people to say, 'You'll grow out of this phase,' but when it comes to being overly concerned with how other people see you, trust me, you will grow out of this phase! By the time you get to your late teens or early twenties, your mind and body will think and feel very differently than they do now and you will be on a much firmer footing than you are now on many fronts.

Above all, though, don't fall into the trap of wrongly thinking there is something abnormal about you if you are still trying to understand your sexual orientation. Rather than criticising yourself for not having the answer by now, I suggest you have as much fun (safely!) as you can in figuring it out!

COMING OUT

Deciding when and how to speak about your sexual orientation is something that heterosexual lads don't have to consider. For example, I didn't have to ponder the possible consequences of my friends or family knowing I'm sexually attracted to girls. When I joined a new football team I didn't have to think about when or how I would tell my teammates I liked girls. The same is true of every other heterosexual man in Ireland. We just don't have to spend any time considering other people's reactions to knowing about this part of our lives.

It can be a different experience for lads who aren't straight. In some ways, it's sad that many young people even have to consider something like this. After all, since straight lads don't have to come out, why should anyone have to? Maybe this will change in years to come and we will all approach every sexual orientation entirely the same way, but this is still an important question for some young people. I'll give you a quick example of what I'm talking about in case you don't understand what I mean.

Frankie (17) told me he was gay in one of our sessions. He said he hadn't told his family about it.

'Do you have to tell my parents what I just told you?' he asked, in a worried voice.

'Well, let me ask you this,' I said. 'If you just told me that you liked a girl, do you think I'd be rushing to the phone to tell them you're straight? Like, "Listen, guys, I've something really serious to tell you here. Stop what you're doing. You should really sit down before I say this – Frankie is straight!"'

'I suppose not,' he said, and smiled with relief.

I explained to Frankie that his sexual orientation was just as important and valid as anyone else's, and that I would provide him with the support he felt he needed to come out to those around him when he felt ready. I asked him why he thought his parents would react negatively, and he didn't really have an answer. Soon he realised that his reasons to be worried were entirely in his own head. His parents had never given any indication in his whole life that they would react with anything other than full support and acceptance in a situation like this. He had read several accounts from people online who had gotten negative reactions and he wrongly assumed it would be the same for him. When he eventually told them himself, he was pleased to learn how wrong he was.

Frankie told them in his own time, when he felt ready, and it went exactly as he would have hoped. His parents said they weren't in any way surprised and were just glad he had reached a point where he was able to talk about it. They were as supportive and accepting of him and his sexuality as they were of his older siblings, all of whom were straight.

For many young people, Frankie's experience is the norm. They spend a lot of time worrying about a negative reaction that never comes. When they come out, they receive nothing but positive comments and everyone just happily moves on with their lives. In fact, I've had some clients who were almost disappointed their parents and friends were so cool and breezy about them talking for the first time about their sexuality.

It's not like this for everyone, however. We can all think of slogans or catchy phrases we've seen on social media about equality, love and relationships, but the reality is that many people suffer discrimination as a result of not being straight. Laws have changed in Ireland, same-sex marriage has been legalised, but there are still people in society who think negatively towards gay people and gay relationships. This is why people are often private and selective about discussing this aspect of themselves.

I'm saying all this to make a fairly obvious point: if you're gay or bisexual, or if you haven't yet settled on any particular word to describe your sexual orientation, it's wise to consider how and when you would like this aspect of yourself to be known by others.

I'll give you some examples of different approaches used by lads I worked with in therapy.

Jason

Jason was 14 and knew he was gay. By the time he was 15, he had told his parents and three of his closest friends. It took him another couple of years to be comfortable with his whole school year knowing, but that was his approach. He needed those few years to grow comfortable with the idea of being openly gay.

Paul

Paul was 18 and was adamant he wasn't going to tell anyone that he was bisexual. A really talented footballer, he was afraid of how his teammates would react, and he didn't want his parents to know. He spoke about his sexuality with me in sessions, but nowhere else, and he kept this up for over two years. Then he gradually started to open up to his closest friends. He needed that time and those sessions to help him become ready to make that next step.

Adam

Adam was 32, and married to a woman. He said he had known he was gay since he was a teenager and was too afraid to come out because he said his family would completely reject him. For him, the cost of people knowing would be too great, so he chose to act as if he were straight for an easier life. He regularly had sex with men but he made sure nobody ever found out. To him, this was his best option.

Liam

Liam's parents and all his friends had known he was gay since he was in his early teens. It never crossed his mind to keep it secret from anyone. He was 17 when he came to see me (the reason he came to therapy had nothing to do with his sexuality). He received nothing but positivity and respect from everyone about this so he couldn't understand why anyone would ever have a problem coming out.

Pete

Even though everyone knew Pete (18) was gay, he never actually came out. He didn't need to. Everyone had just assumed he was gay since he was five or six years old, so no 'announcement' was required when he was a teenager. He was being called gay by classmates and siblings long before he even realised it himself. Pete felt angry that he was denied the chance to decide when others got to learn about this aspect of his life.

As you have probably gathered by now, this is a very personal choice for people to make. What feels right for some lads would feel wrong to others. Some prefer to begin by speaking to trusted friends or supportive parents when they feel ready. Others begin by looking for support online from organisations that offer advice and guidance. Therapists can also provide support to lads who want to chat through their options and help understand the risks and benefits of each one.

It can be a mix of excitement, fear, joy and relief when you're coming out for the first time, but it's a significant step for people to take. The best advice is to go with an approach that you think would work best for you personally, and to remember that coming out isn't a one-time thing. You will only have to do it once with your parents, for example, but you have the option of coming out every time you meet new people and go to new places. After a while, though, this will become less and less of an issue. Not only will you be less concerned by other people's opinions and reactions as you get older, but your level of comfort and understanding towards your sexual orientation will increase. And maybe, just like Frankie, you might look back on the time you spent worrying about this issue and wonder why you worried at all.

SAFETY FIRST

I'm well aware that any chats about safety can often feel like lectures to teenagers. And let's be honest, 'safety' is a topic that doesn't really excite that many people. Most of us want to have fun and enjoy ourselves, so someone banging on about safety is often the last thing we want to hear. However, in the world of sex and relationships, particularly when you're having some of your first experiences, it is vital to grasp the basics of keeping yourself safe. This is particularly the case when you don't have much experience of having sex with other men. Rather than waffle on in a vague way about what I mean, I'll give you a specific example from my therapy room of what can go wrong.

Leo (20) had gone on his own to the house of a man he had met on a gay dating app the previous week. They hadn't even spoken to one another on the phone. The man turned out to be a lot older than he said he was (he had used photos from his younger days on his profile), and from the moment Leo arrived he felt unsafe. He had told the man a few days earlier that he would be comfortable to have sex with him, but Leo immediately regretted this when he got there and wanted to leave. The man overpowered him and raped him. The ordeal lasted about two hours.

The man knew Leo was still private about this sexuality, which made him think he could do what he liked to Leo and get away with it. Since Leo was still uncomfortable with people knowing he was gay, he felt unable to talk to friends about the attack or report it to the police. He had nobody to speak to about this (it took a huge amount of effort for him to make contact with me, eight months later). This wasn't my first experience of working with young gay lads who had been preyed upon by older men.

Myself and Leo did a lot of work together to help him recover from what he had been through and to empower him to live openly, comfortably and safely as a young gay man.

Crimes like this are not unique to the gay community, as I'm sure you're well aware. Obviously, the vast majority of scenarios like this one don't end with people being the victim of violent crime.

The gay scene, however, particularly for younger men, can become hyper-sexual very quickly. In other words, there can be more of an emphasis on sexual encounters than romantic connections. In a world where hook-ups and sexual experiences are many people's primary focus, spending time developing relationships can often be overlooked. So too can the idea of staying safe. Very quickly, it can become all about hook-ups and sexual experiences more than anything else, which can sometimes put people in vulnerable situations. **Remember, you are free to explore or express your sexuality whatever way you choose, but you should always keep an eye on your own safety too.**

SEX AND RELATIONSHIPS — FINDING WHAT WORKS

If you'd rather take the time to get to know someone before being sexual with them, it's important to communicate this to any potential partner. It's perfectly OK to want to develop a deeper connection with someone before you're willing or ready to be intimate with them. You don't have to act as if you're always up for being sexual just because your partner wants it or expects you to want the same. Forget any stereotypes you've heard about how men should think about this (for example, that we should always be up for sex all the time!) and just approach things in ways that feel most comfortable for you. For you, it might be better to slow things down by spending more time speaking and hanging out with lads you like before rushing into sexual situations you feel you're not ready for.

If you'd prefer to seek casual sexual experiences with partners, that's perfectly OK too. **This is your life, remember, and whatever approach you want to take is up to you.** If this is your preference, however, prioritise practising safer sex (see the 'Safer Sex' chapter) and take other safety precautions. Protecting your sexual health and the health of your partners is important, obviously, but so too is ensuring you keep yourself safe. This is sound advice to give any young person, regardless of sexual orientation, but it's particularly needed for people who are drawn to having sexual encounters with random strangers on a casual basis.

The good news is that once you get this part right and take necessary steps around your own safety, all that's left is for you to have as much fun as you possibly can!

SEX IS SEX

As you read through the remaining chapters, you may notice that sexual orientation doesn't get mentioned very much in certain parts. I don't want you thinking that, just because this chapter deals with issues around being gay and bisexual, the rest of the book is just for people who identify as being straight. In other words, if you're gay, I don't want you to think this section is the only section that's relevant to you in this book. As you'll soon find out, the issues I'm going to cover in the remaining chapters are most certainly relevant to you.

Consent, for example, is an issue of paramount importance to individuals and couples of any and all sexualities. We all need to get a handle on it. The need to be aware of how alcohol can impact people's thinking and behaviour is important for everyone too. It's definitely not a message that only straight people should hear. In fact, even non-drinkers would benefit from understanding what happens to someone once they're under the influence of alcohol.

In addition to that, being able to develop, enjoy and end relationships in the healthiest way possible is something that every one of us should understand as well as we can. People of every orientation should read about that. Also, knowing the best ways to keep you and your partner safe from harm is important to us all. And when it comes to porn and the potential impact it can have on how you understand sex, intimacy and pleasure, you'd better believe that it's an area that every young person should understand.

These issues are certainly not limited to people who identify as straight, so whatever your orientation happens to be, make sure you keep reading!

Jack

Jack's parents brought him to see me because they figured he needed someone to talk to. They weren't sure what was bothering him, but they thought he would be more comfortable speaking to an 'outsider' rather than to them. Jack was in fifth year at the time. It took him several sessions to learn to trust me or to speak openly about his own life, but it turned out his parents were right that something personal was bothering him a lot. Jack said he knew he wasn't straight, but wasn't sure after that. He genuinely liked his girlfriend but said he was also attracted to lads. He watched straight porn *and* gay porn, which he found very confusing. He was worried how his friends and teammates would react if they knew. He thought his brothers would treat him differently. He didn't know what his parents would say either, but he thought his girlfriend would be devastated if he told her. Jack seemed to be thinking about everyone else's feelings except his own, and was very critical of himself for being dishonest. Jack used our sessions together to talk openly about this issue and to help him understand and accept himself more. Over time, he started to care less about how to define his sexual orientation, and when he felt ready, he spoke honestly about this to people close to him who he trusted.

I got an email from Jack years later (when he was 21) saying he didn't care about labelling his sexuality anymore. He accepted he was attracted to both men and women, and said he was in a six-month relationship with a fella from Manchester who his family and mates all really liked. He joked that his main problem now was that his boyfriend supported City (Jack follows United!).

Tom

Tom was 17 when his parents brought him to see me. They were concerned that his mood had dipped significantly and they didn't know why. When they left the room, Tom explained what was going on. He said he really fancied one of his best mates in school, Matthew. The problem for Tom was that Matthew was straight, and no matter how many times he brought the topic up with him (which was a lot!), Matthew had no interest in any kind of relationship. The more Matthew said no, the more isolated, hurt and rejected Tom would feel. He couldn't understand that someone he was so close to could be so dismissive of him as a potential boyfriend. Matthew kept repeating that he wasn't gay and that nothing Tom could say was going to change that. It was an important lesson for Tom. As much as it hurt, he had to learn to respect his friend's sexuality, and that constantly making unwanted advances at other people is not appropriate. He started to realise that while he was eager for other people to respect his sexual orientation, he was acting in a way that wasn't showing respect for another person's sexual orientation. Tom realised that despite his own feelings, he needed to accept Matthew the way he was or risk jeopardising their friendship altogether.

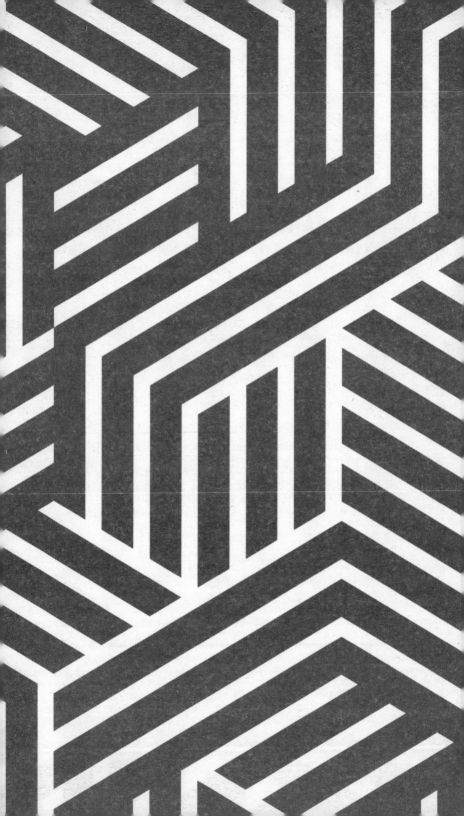

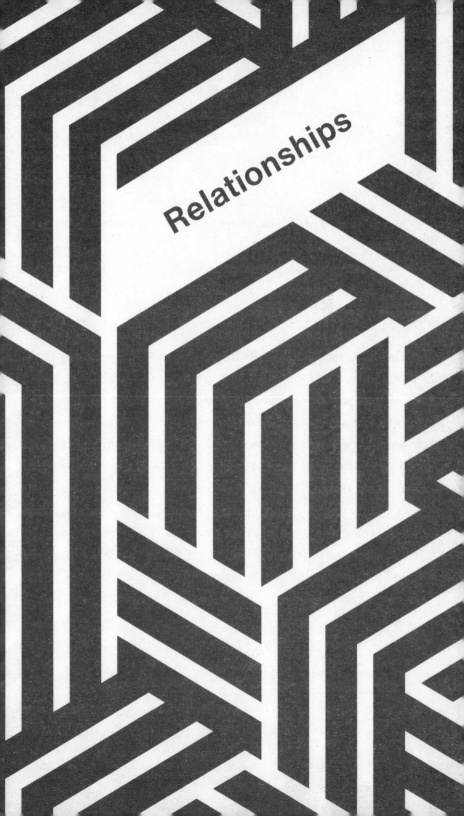

Relationships

I bet you've had loads of guidance from your parents on how to be a good son. I bet you've had loads of input from teachers on how to be a decent student. If you've ever played sport for any length of time then you've had plenty of coaching on how to be a better competitor. There are loads of areas of your life where certain people give you specific guidance, but **where do you get your knowledge on how to behave when you're in a relationship?**

From the movies? From porn? From your parents? From mates? Seriously, where do you get your guidance about this part of your life?

One of the opinions that I hear often from lads in workshops or in my practice is that 'girls are better at relationships than we are'. 'We haven't a clue about all this' is a phrase I hear a lot. Their belief is that girls are better at saying how they feel and better at showing their emotions when it's needed. They're better at getting their way if there's a dispute, and they're better at having the kinds of tricky conversations that sometimes have to be had between partners. This isn't true for everyone, obviously, but each time I hear someone say this, I take it that they're looking for a little help and direction with this stuff themselves. If you think you could also do with some input on the topic of relationships, this chapter is for you.

Let's *not* talk about relationships

Lads weren't given any support about relationships years ago. It just wasn't in our curriculum anywhere in school, and nobody away from school provided any guidance either. I remember people spending hours every week telling me how to be a better footballer but not once did I get any input on being a boyfriend. (I really needed it, as you will tell from reading the next section!)

Today, we're a little better at speaking to teenage lads about relationships, but unfortunately most of the conversations sound like lectures about not behaving badly. Most of the media coverage of teenage behaviour by lads is generally about the times when someone does something really bad. **The more negative stories there are, the more it seems that the only way people speak to teenage lads about relationships is to criticise them or assume the worst.** Adults are generally really good at shaming teenagers who make poor decisions or act inappropriately, but they're not so good at stepping in early enough to have open and frank conversations about some of the issues that arise for young couples.

You're at the stage when relationships are becoming a part of your world. If you're not in one already, I bet you know someone your age who is. Just because topics like sexting and break-ups, for example, can be tricky to discuss, it doesn't mean you should avoid learning about them. The more experience you have yourself, the better you'll be able to work things out on your own, but for now, this chapter will introduce you to some of the things you should watch out for in relationships.

(Just to give you a heads-up, though, there's virtually no chance you'll get through your whole adolescence without making memories that you'll cringe about in later life, but I think you're better off having some information in advance about the scenarios and situations you may soon be facing.)

Me and relationships

I was 10 when I was in my first relationship. We kissed once, and I honestly didn't have a clue what I was at. I remember knowing you were meant to do something particularly impressive with your tongue, so I think I just closed my eyes and launched my mouth in the general direction of her face and hoped for the best. It all happened in front of about six of our friends cheering us on in the wonderfully romantic setting of the church car park. It was over two years before I did anything like that again, but I don't have particularly fond memories of the second one either. This time myself and a girl were kissing behind the school after the local disco had ended. We weren't boyfriend and girlfriend. It was just a one-off thing. I thought it went grand, but a week later her mum rang my mum to tell her I had been touching her daughter's bum and her boobs and she wasn't one bit happy about it. Obviously, I was mortified! I figured I'd just stick to football and stay away from girls from then on.

I was 18 before I lost my virginity, but I stupidly didn't use a condom and was too drunk to remember much of it. My first 'love' was when I was 18, but unfortunately her feelings weren't the same as mine and we didn't last long (she cheated on me with one of my teammates!).

Obviously, relationships are about much more than just kissing and sex, but these are the strongest memories I have. **It's not realistic to expect everything to go perfectly well in this area of your life – that's not how relationships work at all! – but I really hope your own first experiences go a little better than all of mine.**

RELATIONSHIPS

There are many different kinds of relationships. The one you have with your dad is very different than the one you have with your least favourite cousin. The one you have with your best mate is nothing like the one you have with your family pet. You know all this already, but the kinds of relationships I'm talking about in this section are sexual or romantic ones only.

It's worth pointing out that there is no 'normal' age for people to have their first experiences in this area. Everyone has their own path to travel on this one. Many lads your age have no interest in finding a partner or having sexual experiences with anyone just yet. Plenty would really like to meet someone but the opportunity hasn't yet arrived, while there are others who already know what it's like to be someone's partner.

And just to make another obvious point, there are several different ways to describe the kinds of relationships people have with one another that involve sex or romance. I won't list them all now because there are too many. To be honest, though, it doesn't matter how you describe your relationship or how you refer to the person you're with; this section is about some of the issues that may come up for you and your partners. It's also about helping you to tease out for yourself how you would like to behave in a relationship.

INFATUATION, OBSESSION AND BALANCE

I've spoken with lads who are infatuated with the people they fancy, and others who are obsessed with sex. There's a big difference. The ones who are infatuated with certain people spend all their emotional energy thinking about being with them and becoming their boyfriend. They imagine how their life would be so much more delightful if this happened.

Ciaran (18), for example, couldn't stop thinking about Gill, one of the girls in his own group of friends. He loved everything about her appearance and her personality and wanted to message her all the time. They liked loads of the same things and always got on great. He was trying to work up the courage to ask her to his debs. Gill was one of the most popular girls in the area, so he was worried that if he didn't act quickly the chance would pass. His fear was that she'd say no and it would be the end of their friendship.

A HEALTHY RELATIONSHIP IS ONE WHERE BOTH PEOPLE MATTER.

Freddie (19) had a different focus to Ciaran. Freddie was infatuated with sex. He spent his days dreaming about being sexual with girls in any way he could. He didn't have any particular girl in mind who he would like to get together with. His goal was just to have sexual experiences as soon and as often as he could, with as many girls as possible. He had virtually no interest in forming any kind of romantic connection with anyone. He couldn't think of any better way to spend his time than having sex.

Lots of sex education is about imparting information and facts to young people, but there's another important element. It should also get you thinking about what you want for yourself, and what kinds of experiences, relationships and partners you would like to have.

If you're like Ciaran, a lot of your time and energy will be spent on forming and maintaining relationships with people you really like. There will be lots in this chapter that will interest you. If you're like Freddie, and you have more of a focus on sexual experiences than choice of partners, there's plenty here for you too.

There are lots of things to consider if you're hoping to have partners soon or if you're already starting to have relationships. Whether you identify more with Ciaran's approach or Freddie's approach – or you have a different focus entirely – **it's time to start thinking about how you would like to present yourself in this new world.**

SEXUAL DESIRE

It's perfectly normal to want to have sexual experiences in your mid-to-late teens. The old approach to sex education was to shame anyone and everyone who enjoys sex, especially young people. I think it's better to leave that thinking in the past. If being sexual with people is your main focus, that's perfectly fine. It's your life, remember. **However, just like any activity that involves interactions with other people, you've got to keep in mind how your behaviour affects them.** This is certainly the case if we're talking about sexual activity.

I spoke about this a lot with Freddie. He was honest with me about his motives with girls, but he was never honest with them. This wasn't a problem for him, but he was constantly learning that it was a pretty significant problem for many of them. Instead of being upfront about his reluctance to form relationships, he lied about it every time. When he spoke to girls online, he would talk about his hopes of finding someone to go travelling with after he finished college. He told them he wasn't interested in flings in the way that some of his friends were. In fact, he was often critical of men who didn't seem to settle down and fall in love. Pretty much every word out of his mouth was untrue, all designed to trick the girls he was speaking to into thinking he was someone he wasn't. As soon as he was sexual with them in any way, he ghosted them and moved on to someone else. Most of the girls sent messages that made it very clear what they thought of his behaviour.

He never considered the feelings of the girls he was with. In fact, the more he talked about them, the more he made out that he saw them and their bodies as his playthings. It was like his only aim was to ejaculate and he wanted to use them and their bodies to make that happen. However, the more abusive messages he received from the girls he hurt, the more he started to think about the way he was behaving.

Freddie had a choice to make. He could continue as he did, leaving a trail of hurt girls behind him, or he could adopt a more honest approach and cause far less difficulty for himself or anyone else. It took him a while to move to the second option, but after a few bumpy experiences initially, he found that it worked far better for him. He was pleasantly surprised to realise that many girls also wanted sexual experiences and weren't interested or emotionally available for anything more serious.

Like Freddie, every one of us has a choice in how we behave. You're probably younger than he was when I was working with him, but you're at the stage when you can start thinking for yourself what way you'd like to be with other people, whether it's girls or boys you're attracted to. Wanting to have sexual experiences is a perfectly fine and healthy way for you to be, but if your approach is to present yourself as something you are not, it is a sure way of creating a lot of difficulty for others, and also for yourself.

Remember, it's OK not to want a romantic connection with someone. It's OK to want sexual experiences too, so it shouldn't be necessary to present yourself to potential partners as someone you're not.

SEXTING

If sex is your agenda, you'll be trying to create scenarios where sex will happen. Conversations with people you meet online and messages you exchange with people you know will all be shaped by this ultimate goal. And, if your focus is to form a romantic connection with someone, sex is something that may become a feature of your relationship in due course. Either way, sexting is something you may encounter in your future. You may have no experience of this, or no interest in ever doing it, but it's worth discussing it in case it's something you choose to do in years to come.

You are part of one of the first generations of teenagers who have the ability to sext each other using smartphones. If something comes into your head that you'd like to say or send to someone, you can act on it straight away. You can take a picture and send it to anywhere in the world within seconds. You don't have to wait days for your photo to be developed by a chemist like I did, and you don't have to queue outside an internet café for online access. You can text what you like and send it to someone instantly. (Teenagers in the past had to write it in a letter and put it in the post!) **Smartphones remove all that hassle that previous generations had to deal with, but crucially, they also rob you of the 'thinking time' to consider what you're about to do.** You can act on any thought that comes into your head within seconds, which I'm sure you know can be both a good and bad thing!

Just to be clear on what I'm talking about, 'sexting' refers to sending, receiving or forwarding sexually explicit messages and images. There is obviously huge potential to have loads of fun and excitement while sexting, but there are clearly some dangers and downsides to be aware of too. It goes without saying, but I'll say it anyway – this is not an area where you want to run into any difficulties!

When sending an explicit picture of yourself ...

It has become completely normal for people to take pictures of themselves and their friends as they go about their daily lives. Most of us have cameras on our phones so every moment can be captured on film if we act quickly enough. Posting these pictures online and sharing them with others is fairly routine for loads of us too. In other words, sharing images of our lives with others is what many of us do without giving it much thought.

However, when it comes to a picture in which you are nude or partially nude, you really need to think about things very carefully before sending it to anyone. When you're talking about a picture in which someone is nude, an entirely different set of considerations come into play.

Not everyone would be comfortable posting nude photos, obviously. In fact, many people will go through their whole lives without ever being interested in sharing images of themselves with anyone. However, if you're ever in a scenario where you may be thinking about doing this yourself, here are some important points to consider. These suggestions came directly from lads I spoke to who had experience of sexting – both positive and negative – when I asked them what they would tell their younger selves about how to behave in this area.

- Once you press send, you have ZERO control over where it will then go. There is no way of ensuring that the intended recipient will be the only person to see it.

- Ask yourself if you are completely comfortable sending it. If you're not, trust your instinct and don't send it.

- If you're being pressured by someone into sending it against your will, you're dealing with the kind of person who you certainly shouldn't trust with nude images of yourself.

- Spend a minute imagining how you'd feel if your parents, teachers, friends or siblings ended up seeing the image. This should help to focus your mind on making sure this doesn't happen.

- If you and your partner broke up in the near future, how comfortable would you be about them having any images of you? Have you discussed how this will be handled? (If it helps, imagine how you'd feel if an ex from a relationship you really cringe about had some images of you.)

- Are you identifiable in the picture or not? Is your face in it? Being clearly identifiable increases the potential for harm if it is widely circulated without your consent.

- How well do you know the person you're sending it to? How much do you trust them? Do you know if they have ever inappropriately shared images of anyone else, for example?

- How do you know for sure that the image isn't going to be used to blackmail you?

- If you're sending it to someone online, are you 100 per cent sure they are who they say they are? What proof do you have that it's not a fake profile?

You might have read through that list and thought, 'Yeah, they all seem reasonable,' and wonder why anyone could make sloppy mistakes or get things wrong in this area. However, there is one really significant factor: the people doing the sexting are most likely feeling horny at the time! You may have learned this already, but people don't often make sensible, rational decisions when they're sexually aroused. (Remember the bit at the start of this book about what your erection would say if it could speak?!) We can all get carried away in the moment while we're aroused, and make decisions based on what will give us the greatest pleasure in that instant. **In other words, horniness can get in the way of our ability to think straight, so we're a little more vulnerable to behaving in ways we may regret.** This is why going through these considerations now (when presumably you're not feeling horny!) is so important.

I don't like advising people to think of all the things that can go wrong before they do something, especially when it comes to enjoying themselves sexually. Sexting can bring a lot of fun and enjoyment to any relationship. It can be a really exciting way to be sexual with one another, but it's important to be aware of the risks involved.

Even if you really know and trust the person you're sexting, you can still run into difficulty. Images you send to each other can be seen by others without your knowledge or consent, and forwarded or circulated. There are lots of ways this can happen. Phones and social media accounts can get hacked (this happens all the time). Devices can be lost or stolen, as I'm sure you're well aware. Parents often check teenagers' phones, remember, and any one of your friends could go through your phone and see images without you realising it.

All of these are beyond your control, obviously, but they happen all the time. Sexting can be exciting and fun for people who are comfortable getting involved, but you'll pay a potentially high price if your picture is seen by an unintended audience. So, box clever!

When receiving a nude image of someone else …

If someone has sent you a nude image of themselves, they obviously trust you to know how to handle it appropriately. Always assume it's for your eyes only. If they wanted others to see it, they would send it to others themselves. **When receiving a nude image of someone else, you should treat it with the same level of protection and security that you'd treat a picture of yourself.** In other words, do everything you can to ensure it doesn't get into the wrong hands. Remember, it's a photo of a person, not just a photo of a naked (or partially naked) body. Sometimes photos can be seen by others accidentally, but it's a pretty enormous betrayal of trust to deliberately share a nude image of someone else without their agreement. In fact, it's also against the law.

If you know anyone who thinks it's OK or harmless to do this, there are two legal issues you need to make them aware of. (It would be great if you could make them aware of these issues *before* they act!)

First of all, since 2021 it has been a crime under Irish law to share sexual imagery of another person without their consent. It is now known as 'image-based sexual abuse', and anyone found guilty will be considered a sex offender in the eyes of the law and could face prison terms of up to seven years if convicted.

Secondly, anyone under the age of 18 is considered a child in the eyes of the law in Ireland. Any sexual imagery of under-18s is considered child sex abuse material. If you send or share an explicit image of anyone under 18 you are guilty of distributing child sex abuse material and could face criminal prosecution.

I'll give you one example which explains how seriously this issue is taken. Harry (17) got the shock of his life when he was called to the principal's office. His parents were there, sitting next to the vice-principal, his year master and two Gardaí. Harry had shared images of his ex-girlfriend (16) with friends who forwarded them to loads of other people. The girl's parents found out and reported him to the Gardaí. They confiscated his phone, which had other images of his ex and some other girls of that age. When we started our first session together, he was facing charges of possessing and distributing child sex abuse material and expulsion from school. His parents were mortified and furious with him, and Harry genuinely wanted his life to be over. I can only imagine how hurtful it was for the girl involved.

Even if you put aside the legal issues, sharing imagery of someone else without their consent is a pretty horrendous thing to do to them. In fact, it's very hard to think of many other things in relationships that are as hurtful or harmful as this. People like Harry learn the hard way how serious this is. The reason I've told you about his experience is to help you learn too.

When someone forwards you a pic of someone else

Delete it immediately! That's the main advice that comes from lads who have been in this position before. It's exactly what Harry's friends wished they had done. There are no scenarios where it is OK for you to have a nude pic of someone else on your phone without their knowledge or permission. If the person in the picture didn't send it to you themselves, assume they don't want you to see it.

Of course, you're of an age where you make your own decisions around this stuff. You could avoid ever sending a picture of yourself to anyone, and you can make it clear to partners that you'd prefer not to receive one. Whatever personal choices you make on this one, just remember that all intimate pictures, whether you are in them or not, should be treated with the utmost respect at all times. **Sexting is just like many other aspects of sexual activity – if you take the necessary safety precautions to limit the risks to you and your partners, all that's left is to concentrate on having as much fun and enjoyment as possible.**

WHAT'S A HEALTHY RELATIONSHIP?

If I asked you to describe a healthy relationship, what would you say? I don't mean describe your ideal relationship or your favourite kind of partner. I'm not asking you to list off the things you'd like to do with your partner either. What I'm looking for is a description of a relationship that's healthy. If I asked you to do this, would you know where to start?

There are loads of ways to answer a question like this, but it's really important you understand what I mean by healthy. It doesn't mean being happy all the time. It doesn't mean you never disagree or break up. It doesn't mean living happily ever after together, either. **A healthy relationship is one where both people matter.** It's where both people feel like their voices are heard, their opinions matter and their preferences are taken into account. If there's a bump in the road (which happens in almost every relationship at some point!), they're able to work together to find a way round it. It doesn't mean always letting the other person have their way. A healthy relationship is one where both people can talk, hear and negotiate with care and respect.

You learn the most about relationships from having real-life experiences of your own. I could try to explain heartbreak, for example, but you'll only truly understand it when you go through it. I could talk about how great it is to be in love, but if you've never experienced it yourself you mightn't fully get it. However, there are some things you can learn without having to wait to experience them for yourself.

When I ask lads in schools to describe healthy relationships, the most common replies I get are descriptions of behaviour that shows that things are really *un*healthy. In other words, they list off ways that people shouldn't treat one another or give examples of situations that are going badly wrong. It's usually things they've experienced when they were in relationships themselves or things they've seen or heard about from others. Here are the most common answers they'd give to describe scenarios where things have gotten unhealthy between a couple:

- If one person won't let the other go on holiday with their mates (on a girls'/lads' holiday).

- If one person knows the other is being unfaithful, but likes them too much to break up.

- If one person is constantly controlling or criticising the other one.

- If one person insists on going through the other person's phone to keep tabs on them.

- If they are constantly fighting and ignoring one another for long spells.

- If one person is just using the other for sex but the other person thinks it's more serious.

- If one person doesn't trust the other to go on a night out without them being there.

- If one of you tries to control who the other person can be friends with.

- If one person pressures the other to send pics when they know they don't want to.

It's possible to add countless other examples to this list. In fact, you could fill a whole book with the many unhealthy ways people could behave in a relationship. These are just the most common suggestions given in the workshops I did. What's important here is that you learn to notice for yourself the many different red flags that can appear at various points in a relationship. Remember, your red flags may differ from other people's, and they may even differ from your partner's list, but take it from me: it's really not a good idea to ignore red flags if they start to appear!

BREAK-UPS

If you stay single for your entire life, you'll never have to find out what it's like to go through a break-up. Where's the fun in that, though? Staying together with the first person you kiss for your entire life is the only other way to avoid a break-up, but what are the chances of that happening? Not many people give this much thought, but with the exception of the person you're in a relationship with on the day you die, you will break up with every partner you have throughout your life. In fact, I'd say there's a pretty high probability (close to 90 per cent would be my guess!) that the relationship you're in when you're 18 years old will not be a lifelong one. In other words, breaking up is something that practically everyone will go through at some point.

You might see this as a negative or gloomy statement, but I don't see it that way at all. The quality of a relationship isn't judged solely by how long it lasts or how soon it ends. And just because it ends doesn't mean it was a failure, or that it didn't work, or that it should never have happened. Rather than pretend that relationships never end, I think it's better to talk about break-ups in a way that is actually useful.

It may surprise you to realise that break-ups don't *have* to be upsetting and hurtful. They *can* be, but they don't *have* to be. Despite what you might have seen in movies, ex-partners don't *have* to spend time annoying, slagging, ignoring or hurting one other. Even though you might have real-life examples much closer to home of people being awful to one another during and after break-ups, you shouldn't think that this is the way it's meant to be for everyone. Yes, break-ups *can be* upsetting, painful and sad, but that doesn't mean they can't be healthy too.

You have no control over how your (ex-)partner is going to handle it, but here's how to play your part in the break-up being healthy.

Dos

If you have made the decision to break up, say it to your partner's face, in a place that's private. (If the relationship has been abusive, however, it may be better to do it over the phone or by text to avoid an aggressive or violent confrontation.) There are no rules about how long these conversations should last or how much or little you should say. It's OK to say your feelings have changed if that's the truth. You just have to be honest and, ideally, thoughtful. If your partner is the one who wants to end it, you have to accept their decision. **Your feelings do matter, obviously, but they don't matter more than your partner's right to end things if that's how they feel.** In time, you can both decide whether you'd like to remain friends or whether it's better not to stay in touch. This can be a decision you work out between you both. If you've both been very public about your relationship on social media, for example, you can decide as a couple how you would like to handle the break-up on social media too. You can choose whether to remove pics of one another from your profiles, for example. If you both hang out in the same places, you can decide to deliberately avoid going there for a while, or work out ways to keep out of each other's social spaces. If you have the same friends, you can decide together what to tell them about the break-up. In summary, you can treat your (ex-)partner with the same level of decency during the break-up as I presume you showed them when you were together.

Don'ts

The list of ways to be a dick in this situation is endless, but I'll name the obvious ones. Don't break up with someone on social media. Don't send your mate to do it for you. Don't deliberately hook up with someone in front of them just so they'll break up with you (my mate once did this!). Don't share any nude pics of your ex with anyone. Don't spread stories that would hurt or embarrass them. Don't keep messaging them if they've asked you not to. Don't give them hope you'll get back together if you have no intention of it. Don't post snotty remarks about them online. Don't share information with others that they told you in confidence. Don't be intentionally rude or hurtful if you meet each other when you're out, and don't think you have a say in who they should or shouldn't choose as their next partner. **In summary, don't act in a way that spoils everything you ever had between you.**

Most people would never consider any of these behaviours, but the real test comes when we get hurt. Julian (17), for example, would have laughed at a list like this if I showed it to him while he was with his ex, but everything changed because he was so hurt by how they broke up. After a few sessions speaking about the break-up, he was able to talk about how upset he really felt. Up until then, however, he was constantly slagging his ex-girlfriend to their friends and sending her insulting and hurtful messages, because he thought that was what you were meant to do in these kinds of situations. After a while, we worked out that he found it a lot easier to be angry than to be sad, which was why he spent his time criticising her instead of admitting he was gutted they broke up. It was easier for him to act like he hated her than to feel sorry for himself. He was really hurt and felt really rejected, something he had never felt before. His pride was hurt also, because she chose to be with someone else quite soon after they broke up. Julian needed a lot of coaching and support on how to deal with this break-up because it was his first experience. He came to realise it was healthy for him to feel upset because he liked her so much, but it was very unhealthy to express those feelings as anger and resentment.

Break-ups can be very amicable when both people feel the same, but they can be very tricky if one person doesn't want the relationship to end. It's much easier if you make the decision yourself, but it can be hard to take if your partner is the one who ends things with you. It's not possible, however, to be in a relationship with someone who doesn't want to be there, so you don't have a choice.

Nobody gets this right every time, but going into every break-up with the intention of doing things in a healthy way is the best approach.

Lessons from the therapy room

Brian

Brian (19) came to see me on his own to talk about a problem he was having with his girlfriend, Nina. They had been together for over two years but he wanted to break up with her. He had tried twice to tell her how he felt, but each time Nina said she would hurt herself if he went through with it. He felt completely trapped. He didn't want to hurt her, and he certainly didn't want her to hurt herself, but he really didn't want to stay in the relationship. Brian hadn't told any of his family or friends about his situation. He thought something as serious as this should be kept a secret. His friends were also Nina's friends so he thought he couldn't speak to them. However, the more Brian spoke to me about his situation, his feelings and his options, the clearer he became on what he felt he should do. He realised he was being emotionally manipulated by Nina and that it had become a very unhealthy relationship. He didn't find it easy talking about personal stuff like this, but he felt he needed to say it to someone. It took him several sessions to tease out what he was going to do, but he was realising the hard way that staying silent about something like this wasn't the right thing to do.

Alan

Alan (18) was brought to see me by his parents to help him with his anxiety. As soon as his parents left the room, he explained the root cause of his constant feelings of worry, anxiety and fear. The previous summer, he had sent nude pictures of himself to a girl he had met online. Within 24 hours, however, he realised he had made a huge mistake. It turns out he was wrong to have completely trusted the total stranger he had just met online. He was contacted by an anonymous social media account (which was deleted shortly after) and sent a link to a website that had posted his pictures that day. His face was identifiable in the images. The pictures were taken down shortly after this, but he lived in constant fear ever since that they would reappear online somewhere, that someone he knew would see them, or that someone would make an attempt to blackmail him. Every time he received a notification on his phone, he would panic. And because he was so embarrassed about it all, he felt he couldn't tell the Guards, his friends, his family or his girlfriend, so he had been suffering this entirely alone for all this time. I helped him to manage his anxiety levels better over the following few months. For Alan, it was the toughest way to learn an important lesson about the need to treat photos of yourself with extreme care.

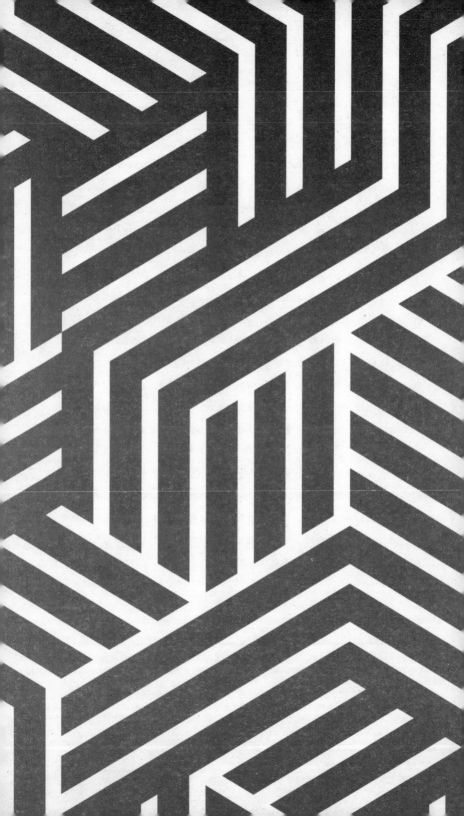

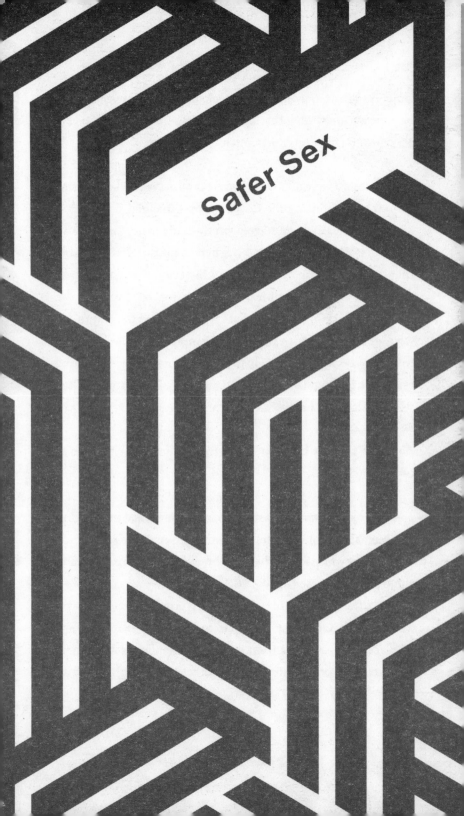

Safer Sex

Unless you've been living under a rock for the last few years, you'll be fully aware by now that diseases, viruses and infections are spread among the human population every day.

The advice we were all given to protect ourselves and each other from infection during the Covid-19 pandemic had a significant impact on where we could go, who we could meet, and how we could act. Every single one of us had to face up to the reality that we were at risk of catching an infection that could cause significant health difficulties, even death, for ourselves or those around us. It didn't matter where we lived or who we were, we were all presented with the same dilemma – were we prepared to act in ways that would help to protect ourselves and our loved ones from getting sick? Or instead, would we do whatever suited us and just hope that we stayed clear of trouble?

These are the very same questions to consider when it comes to our sexual health.

Taking precautionary measures to limit the spread of Covid-19 was seen as common sense. The message was quite straightforward – once you're aware there's a threat of infection, you should act to protect yourself against it. And the more you act to protect yourself, the greater protection you are providing to those you interact with. Of course, it was up to each of us to decide how we'd act, but the advice from public health officials was simple and direct – protect yourselves to protect each other!

The same principle is at play when it comes to your sexual health. Learning about how STIs (sexually transmitted infections) can be transmitted, for example, is just like being taught how Covid-19 can be spread. The more informed you are, the more informed your decisions will be. Supporting you to make more informed decisions in manging your sexual health is one of the primary aims of this book and it's the main focus of this chapter. You can also check out the Appendix (page 209) for more detailed information on how STIs are spread.

This section is about two main topics – protection and contraception. Just to be absolutely clear: **when I say protection, I'm talking about behaviour aimed at protecting you and your partners from acquiring an STI. When I say contraception, I'm talking about measures people can take to prevent pregnancy.**

Let's *not* talk about safer sex

You may not know this, but previous generations of teenagers were given virtually no support or information about safer sex or how to avoid unplanned pregnancies. My parents, and possibly your parents too, were given no education about the importance of sexual health or how to keep themselves safe from catching STIs (apologies for planting the image in your mind of your parents actually having sex!). For a variety of reasons, the approach back then was to keep the conversation around sex as straightforward and simplistic as possible.

The messaging was clear – sex was only for men and women who were married; sex within marriage was to happen for the purposes of getting pregnant. Since people were expected to wait until they were married to have sex, and only have sex with that one person for their entire lives, there was no real reason to acknowledge all the different diseases and infections that people carry with them and can pass on to others when they have unprotected sex with different partners.

There was no acknowledgement that loads of people had no intention of waiting until they were married before having sex, others had no interest in getting married, others wanted to be intimate with sexual partners across the genders, some had no desire to become parents, and plenty of couples had no interest at all in continually getting pregnant throughout their marriage.

Since all of those situations were ignored, there was no reason to even mention condoms, never mind explain why they should be used or how to use them. **In fact, it was illegal to buy condoms in Ireland right up until 1978, the year before I was born, and it wasn't until 1985 that it became possible to buy condoms without a prescription from a GP.**

In Ireland today, condoms are on sale in almost every supermarket and pharmacy in the country. If you're too uncomfortable to buy them over the counter, as many people are, you can just order them online. Information about sexual health and the dangers of unprotected sex has never been more available to teenagers. So, compared to previous generations, you've got it pretty lucky on this one. Books like this wouldn't have been written for lads your age in the past. Once you've read this chapter, you'll be fully briefed on the many ways of keeping you and your partners safe throughout your relationships.

Me and safer sex

I don't remember having any conversation with anyone when I was a teenager about safer sex. I knew what condoms were, obviously, but I can't recall any lessons in school about why they should be used or how to use them correctly. In fact, other than a brief reference to them during Junior Cert biology class, I don't remember condoms even being mentioned. When I first had sex, I didn't use one. I was very drunk at the time and it didn't even cross my mind. The girl I was with didn't mention it, so I figured if she was OK with it, I should be too. That was my attitude in those early years – if my partner didn't insist on it, I wouldn't use one.

It sounds weird now when I look back, but it was like I let my partners decide how safe we were going to be, rather than having any say or taking any responsibility for this decision myself. I didn't think I could ever ask a girl if she was on the Pill either. I know this sounds really odd, but I didn't think it was my place to ask something so personal of someone else. Other than condoms, the Pill was the only form of contraception I heard about, but I was always pretty awkward talking about this stuff.

I'm telling you this because I don't want to give the false impression that I never made any poor decisions in this area myself. I'm not in a position to lecture anyone or pretend as if I always did the right thing. Lots of us make decisions we really regret in this area, but often it's too late by the time we realise how flawed our thinking was. However, it's often from making mistakes that we learn important lessons. This chapter is aimed at passing those lessons on to you.

Personal Responsibility

You might not remember this, but there was a time when your parents did everything for you. A simple task like brushing your teeth, for example, was beyond you. If they didn't do it, it wouldn't get done because you were too young to do it yourself. The list of things that parents and adults do for young children and teenagers is endless, but there is always an unspoken agreement that certain help won't be provided forever. As you grow, you're expected to take over these responsibilities yourself. Brushing your teeth, for example, is a service I bet your parents no longer provide for you, and the list of things you do for yourself is now bigger than ever. In other words, you've got more responsibility for yourself than ever before.

WHEN IT COMES TO PROTECTING YOURSELF, YOU'RE THE ONE IN THE DRIVING SEAT.

Just as taking personal responsibility to brush your teeth regularly to ensure good dental hygiene and fresh breath is important as a teenager, so it is when it comes to your sexual health. Your parents aren't responsible for this one. You may be fortunate enough to belong to a family where information and guidance about sex and sexuality are available, but when important decisions need to be made, you'll be the one making them. **When it comes to protecting yourself from the unwanted consequences of any kind of sexual activity, always remember that you're the one in the driving seat.** The consequences of things going wrong will be on you, so taking the steps to help avoid that happening should be on you too. You're too old now to act as if it's anyone else's job but yours (especially if you think you're too young to be a dad!).

JOINT RESPONSIBILITY

Having just told you about the value of personal responsibility, I hope it doesn't sound like I'm contradicting myself if I now tell you about the importance and benefits of joint responsibility too. Before this gets confusing in any way, let me first explain what I mean.

When it comes to relationships, there is often no absolute 'right' or 'wrong' way of doing things. For example, if you both go to the cinema together, who gets to decide on what you see? If you go out for a meal together, what's the right way for you both to act when the bill arrives? If you both want to do different things on the same night, what's the correct way of deciding what you end up doing together? There is no 'right' or 'wrong' way because every couple has their own way of working through each of these situations.

The answers to these questions can usually only be found by couples discussing their options with one another. Once they're both aware of their options and how they both feel about their choices, they can work together to come up with a plan they're both happy with. In other words, having realised that they are both going to be impacted by the outcome, they work together.

The same approach works really well when it comes to having safer sex together. **The more you talk with one another about the options you have together, the greater chance you'll have of getting things right as a couple.** Remember, you'll both be impacted by an unplanned pregnancy or if one of you has an STI, so taking a joint approach to protecting yourselves is the way to go.

This would be a good time to remind you of what I said about erections and sexual arousal in the opening chapter. It would be very wise to have this conversation before either of you have reached a state of arousal, otherwise your decisions could be made on the basis of your sexual urges. Practical and sensible thinking often takes a backseat when we're aroused, and we often ignore what we know are the best decisions. As I'm sure you understand by now, this is a policy that can land you both in a lot of trouble.

KNOWLEDGE IS POWER

Just like drivers are supposed to have a good understanding of the rules of the road, sexually active people should know about the many different methods of protection and contraception that are available to everyone. **Knowing how to effectively use condoms, for example, is as important as knowing the colours on a traffic light.** You may think it's enough to turn to friends or partners for pointers on how to avoid pregnancies, but without realising it, they may give you advice or guidance that is either misleading or inaccurate. This is one area where you should really make sure you get the right information, so that's what this section is all about.

Is this section for me?

Most lads your age have no desire to become parents any time soon. I certainly didn't when I was a teenager. If that's how you feel, and you hope to become sexually active soon, this section is for you. In fact, regardless of whether you ever want to become a parent in the future, I'm going to assume you're not mad on the idea of getting something like genital warts along the way. If that's the case, and I'd be pretty confident it is, this section is definitely for you.

Just to be absolutely clear on what we're talking about here, I'll say it again: 'protection' is the term I'm using to describe ways people can guard against catching or spreading STIs, and 'contraception' is all about measures people can take to prevent pregnancy. They all come under three different headings:

- Single-use (such as condoms)

- Daily dose (such as the Pill)

- Long-acting (such as the Coil, which can last for years once it's inserted in a woman's body)

I'll run through the options for emergency contraception also, but keep in mind the concept of *dual protection* as you read through this section – this is where couples ensure they take steps to protect themselves against both STIs *and* unplanned pregnancy.

CONTRACEPTION

There are many different types of contraception. They work by preventing a sperm and an egg from connecting in a variety of ways *if* they are used correctly and consistently. I'll take you through some of the most common methods available, and I'll outline the advantages and disadvantages that come with them all. When you become sexually active and you want to avoid an unplanned pregnancy, this is the information you will need.

Abstinence

This is a 100 per cent effective approach. Abstinence is the term we use to describe a situation where a person chooses not to have sex. **To put it bluntly, there's no better way to avoid getting pregnant than to avoid having sex.** It's free, obviously, so there is no financial cost involved. Anyone can try it, and if you don't like how it's going, you can adopt a different approach any time you like. If you stick to this, pregnancy will not be a possibility in your relationship. It's also an ideal option for those who don't feel like they are ready for a sexual relationship. People often assume that lads are always keen to have sex as soon as possible and as often as possible, but we know that's not the case with everyone. If that's you, this approach will slot in perfectly with your lifestyle. This approach, however, would be very challenging for people who enjoy having sex or who wish to experience sex with their partners.

Condoms

Most people know what condoms are and what they're for. The good news is they're widely available and you don't need a prescription from a GP to buy them. There are no known medical side effects of using condoms (unless you've a latex allergy – in which case non-latex condoms should be used), they're easy to carry with you, and they also protect you and your partners from the spread of infections. However, not everyone is aware of how to use them correctly. Here's a step-by-step guide to doing it right.

STEP 1

First of all, it's important to check the expiry date on the packet, and also, check there's a quality mark (CE/Kite) somewhere on the packet too. Once you have both of these, you have a usable condom.

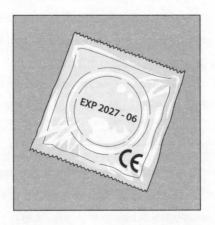

STEP 2

It's important to be careful opening the packet to ensure you don't accidentally damage the condom inside. If you rush this part, you may tear the edge of the condom, meaning it will no longer work effectively. This is why it's no harm to have a spare one with you just in case.

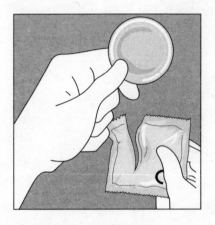

STEP 3

Wait until the penis is fully erect before putting on the condom. Ensure there is no air in the tip of the condom before it is rolled onto the penis. This can be done easily enough by holding the tip together between two fingers to remove any air that's already inside.

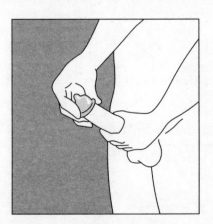

STEP 4

Then roll the condom to the base of the penis, checking to make sure there is no air creating a 'bubble' at the top. If there's a bubble here, there's a good chance the condom will rip during intercourse.

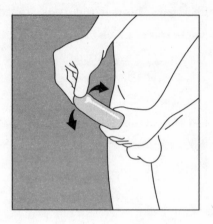

STEP 5

There are two things to keep in mind when removing the condom after use. Firstly, when you are 'pulling out', hold onto the base of the condom to ensure it stays on your penis. Secondly, remember that it's better to do this while your penis is still erect to minimise leakage (men generally lose their erections after ejaculation, so don't hang about!).

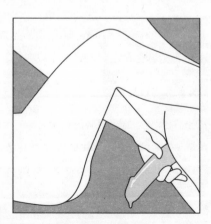

OPTIONS FOR FEMALES

In terms of taking steps to prevent pregnancy, those are the top two options available to men – you either don't have sex or use a condom when you do. The list of options available to females is a lot longer, so I'll run you through them now. You might already be thinking there's no point in reading on, but think again. Even though these methods can only be used by females, if you're planning on being in relationships with women this is the kind of information that would be useful to know. **Remember, you will both have to share in the responsibility of an unplanned pregnancy, so learning as much as you can about how to avoid that is the right way to go.** It's also important to be mindful of the side effects that hormonal contraception can cause, such as irregular bleeding and acne, so it can take a little while to find the most suitable method.

Female condoms

Lots of people don't even know that female condoms exist, but just like male condoms, these are widely available and don't require a prescription. They can be inserted into the girl's vagina up to 8 hours before she has sex. They're not suitable for girls who have an allergy to latex, and they should never be used along with male condoms – it's either one or the other! Just like male condoms, they require a little practice to use correctly.

The Pill

This is one of the most popular and widely used contraceptives in Ireland. In addition to protecting against pregnancy, it can help to reduce PMT (pre-menstrual tension) and period pain. It offers no protection against STIs, however, so it's strongly recommended you wear a condom also to help protect you both when you have sex. There are different kinds of Pill, and they work in different ways, so your partner may have to try more than one type to find the one that works best for them.

Injectable contraception

Using this method, your partner would get an injection from a healthcare professional approximately every twelve weeks. This is an option for girls who don't want to take a pill every day, but just like the Pill, it offers no protection against the spread of infection.

The Coil

In this method, a small device is placed into your partner's womb by a doctor. There are two options here – one is the IUD, which is a small copper and plastic device that lasts between five and ten years, while the other is the IUS, a small plastic device which can last up to five years. They work in different ways, but they're both effective as soon as they're inserted. Just like the other methods aside from condoms, however, they offer no protection against the spread of infection.

Contraceptive implant

If your partner goes with this method, a small flexible rod will be inserted under the skin of her upper arm. It has to be inserted by a doctor, is effective for three years, and can also help to reduce painful periods. Like the other methods aside from condoms, it offers no protection against the spread of infection.

Contraceptive patch

This method involves wearing a patch, similar to a plaster, every day for three weeks, followed by one patch-free week. Many girls prefer this to having to remember to take a pill each day. It requires a prescription from a GP. It is visible on the skin, and is usually a little more expensive than the Pill. Like the other methods, with the exception of condoms, it offers no protection against the spread of infections.

Vaginal ring

In this method, your partner would insert a small, flexible ring into her vagina and leave it for three weeks before removing it. A week later, she will need to insert a new one. Each ring provides contraception for a month, so she won't have to do anything else once it is inserted. It doesn't protect against the spread of infections, however, so using a condom along with this method is advisable.

SUMMARY

Just to recap, **if you and your partner want to avoid an unplanned pregnancy, you're not short of options.** Once you are both clear that you are ready to be sexually active and you wish to avoid pregnancy and any STIs, you will be required to take certain steps to protect yourselves and each other. In addition to ensuring you use a condom every time you have sex, your partner has the following list of options to consider:

- **She can insert a condom into her vagina (if not using a male condom).**

- She can take the Pill each day.

- She can get a hormone injection every three months.

- She can have a device inserted into her womb.

- She can have a rod implanted into her arm.

- She can wear a patch.

- She can insert a vaginal ring.

Regardless of your choices or behaviour, you have now gone past the point where you can claim to be ignorant on these issues. You've enough information to go on now. You know the risks, and you know how to guard against them. However, if despite all that, you find yourself in a scenario where you require emergency contraception, you do have options then too.

EMERGENCY CONTRACEPTION

Other than abstaining from sex altogether, there is no way to guarantee you can avoid unplanned pregnancy. **The fact is that accidents do happen, and some methods, even when used correctly, can let you down**. There are other times, though, when people have unprotected sex and are in need of emergency protection as soon as possible. If a man ejaculates inside a woman without any form of contraception being used, and pregnancy is something the couple wish to avoid, they do have options but they have to move fast.

There are different choices for different situations, but it's important you know what they are. Like earlier, you might think this section isn't for you because you're not the one who has to take the contraception. But you can only be supportive to your partner if you're aware of the options, so it's important to have an understanding of what they are.

First of all, a pharmacist is available for a private consultation to explain the situation and discuss the options (every pharmacy has a private space for discreet conversations between customers and staff). You could talk to your local GP or visit a family planning clinic in your area if you'd prefer. Medical card holders can get emergency contraception free. There are loads of websites where you can get advice in these situations, but it's better to speak directly to medical professionals to ensure you get the right information.

The three-day pill

As the name suggests, this pill can be used in the first three days after sex. It's often referred to as the morning-after pill, and it is 99 per cent effective if taken within 12 hours of unprotected sex. It is less effective on day two or day three. It will be even less effective if your partner has already taken it earlier in the same menstrual cycle. It's available directly from pharmacists without a prescription for over-17s and usually costs around €25.

The five-day pill

This works similarly to the three-day pill, but it can be effective for up to five days after unprotected sex (hence the name!). It can be up to 99.5 per cent effective, but it should be taken as soon as possible. It's also available in pharmacies without prescription to over-17s, but it can cost around €30. If you think this is a little on the expensive side, you should know that compared to the price of parenthood, it's a bargain!

TAKING RISKS

I'm pretty sure you know this already, but some people tend towards risky behaviour more than others. Even within your own family or group of friends, you probably saw a number of different ways to respond to the threat of catching Covid-19.

Some people took every necessary precaution, and didn't think for a second to stray from public health guidelines. Others may have been a little more relaxed, and changed their behaviour day to day depending on their mood.

You may have known some people – and maybe you're one of them yourself – who ignored everything they were advised to do and just did their own thing from day one. I'm not going to mention Covid-19 again, but just like people have different attitudes to following public health guidelines, people also have their own ways of responding to advice on sexual health.

Adolescence is a time for a lot of new experiences, but it is also a stage of life when risk-taking and challenging authority are common for many people. So, when it comes to following advice from adults about how to avoid risks, many teenagers simply switch off. **There's no doubt that sometimes risk-taking can be exciting, but this is one area where taking chances can have lifelong consequences for those involved.**

Before I go on, it's worth pointing out that a huge amount of fun and sexual pleasure can be had without engaging in penetrative sex. There are so many ways for couples to be intimate with one another that don't involve any of the risks discussed in this section. (However, penetration is not the only way STIs can be transmitted.) Obviously, you would avoid the risk of an unplanned pregnancy if you chose to abstain from sex for the time being, and you'd significantly reduce your exposure to potential infections. So if you feel that having penetrative sex isn't the right choice for you now or any time in the future, remember this doesn't mean you'll be depriving you or your partners of enjoyable and satisfying experiences with one another.

In this section, I'll cover a lot of the reasons and excuses young people give for not following advice in this area. It's so important you learn how to protect yourself, so I think it's worth going through each excuse just to highlight why it would be wrong to start thinking that any of them made sense. These are the most common responses I hear from risk-taking young people when they discuss their sexual behaviour in an open and honest way.

Not using condoms when you have sex
REASON 1: *'What are the chances of anything bad happening? Virtually nil!'*
Many young people can't imagine bad things happening to them.

They're convinced they'll just never get caught out, no matter how they behave. They're really positive and hopeful and spend little or no time thinking about things that can go wrong. This attitude can be really helpful in lots of areas, but it's definitely not helpful when it comes to decisions about condoms. For people who think this way, it often means they'll take minimal precautionary measures because they don't even consider that things might not work out the way they want.

It's sometimes a personality trait, but it's often to do with being an adolescent – when risk-taking and challenging authority are really common. Whatever the reason, however, this is a pattern of thinking that causes huge distress for many in this particular area. Always use a condom!

REASON 2: *'My partner didn't ask me to wear one, so obviously I don't need to wear one.'*
This is just as reckless as deciding it's OK not to wear a seatbelt in a car just because the driver didn't mention it. Many lads think this way (I did too!). They interpret their partner's silence as a sign that a condom isn't needed, but it's a strategy that makes no sense. It hands over total responsibility for your sexual health to your partner, as if you've no say on the issue.

This is a particularly dangerous way to think if you don't know your partner's history. Think about it – if all you know about them is that they don't ask their partners to wear condoms during sex, you should definitely not be following their lead on this one. Either they don't know the risks or they're deliberately ignoring the risks. Whatever their reason, this is not a decision you should allow others to make on your behalf.

REASON 3: *'I'll just pull out so there's no need to wear one.'*
This is a really common one. This approach won't protect you from contracting an STI anyway, which should concern you, obviously. However, it won't offer protection against an unplanned pregnancy either – so it's a total failure as a strategy. What some people don't realise is that before a man ejaculates, semen can come from his penis and enter into the woman's vagina without either of them realising it – which can obviously lead to pregnancy.

The message on this one is fairly simple and easy to understand – unless you're hoping the sex will lead to pregnancy, wear a condom!

REASON 4: *'Sex feels better without one.'*
This is like people saying that seatbelts make a drive in a car less comfortable, or that wearing a helmet on a motorbike ruins the experience. Even if you thought these things, it would be unbelievably stupid to travel in a car or on a motorbike without using either.

If you are concerned that protecting yourselves in this way may lessen the sensation or enjoyment of sex, it's worth remembering that condoms come in so many different varieties, flavours and textures. You could have a load of fun experimenting with condoms that allow for extra sensation for you both, so shop around!

REASON 5: *'I generally don't have one with me.'*

It makes zero sense that somebody would not have a condom with them if there was a possibility of a sexual encounter. That's like going to play a match and not bringing football boots. Just like cash, your phone or the keys of your house, a condom should be something you always have on you, just in case, when you're sexually active. Think about it – deciding not to have a condom with you in scenarios where sex is a possibility just increases the possibility of you not having sex, because your partner may be serious about their sexual health and avoiding an unplanned pregnancy.

Always keep this phrase in mind when it comes to having condoms with you at all times – it's better to have them and not need them than to need them and not have them!

Not bringing a condom with you when you go out

REASON 1: *'I'm not expecting or planning a sexual encounter of any kind.'*

This is sound reasoning, but you may at this stage be aware that sexual encounters aren't things that always come with several days' warning. Spontaneous, unplanned, impulsive encounters happen all the time, especially where alcohol is involved. If you're sexually active, it's always better to be prepared. Nobody can claim that carrying condoms is a hardship of any kind given how small they are, so the argument for leaving them at home just doesn't stack up. The more nights out you have and the more you witness what happens around you, the more you'll appreciate that what happens on nights out can be very hard to predict in advance. You'll be prepared for any sexual scenario that unfolds if you're carrying some condoms.

REASON 2: *'Even if I meet someone, we're hardly going to be having sex tonight.'*
Many people would think this. It reflects a view that sex is something that comes later in a relationship or that your sexual desires can easily be ignored at all times. Many people think this way. However, there are occasions, especially when drink is involved, when people act in ways they never would when they're sober. Many people, particularly people who have ever been drunk, can sometimes look back in bemusement at how alcohol impacts their behaviour. So, while it's understandable to think you'll stick to your plans when you're on a night out, you may start to look at your options differently once alcohol is involved.

It is no hassle at all having a condom with you, but not having one when you need it could really be a problem.

REASON 3: *'I'm just not that good at planning ahead.'*
Lots of people are like this. They're spontaneous and just live 'in the moment'. They scoff at the idea that you'd be able to predict the future or plan for it in any way. If you're like this, then you've got even more of a reason to ensure you have a condom with you.

It's the impulsive and spontaneous people who particularly need to have condoms!

REASON 4: *'If I don't have one with me, I won't have to use one!'*
Some lads think this way, hoping that not having a condom increases their chances of having unsafe sex (this is for those who don't like wearing them). It's like deliberately forgetting your PE gear at school to make sure you won't have to join in. However, not having a condom just increases the possibility of you *not* having sex because your partner may take their sexual health seriously. Remember this simple line – unsafe sex should only be happening between partners who wish to get pregnant.

Not asking your female partner if she's using contraception

REASON 1: *'I didn't know her well enough to ask.'*
This generally refers to more casual hook-ups rather than couples who have been seeing one another for a while. Some people think this isn't something you can or should ask a girl who you've just met. However, if you're in a scenario where you are about to have sex with her, you've definitely reached the point where you 'know her well enough' to ask a question as relevant as this one.

This is not one of those issues where it's better to assume the answer – so you have to ask the question. If a pregnancy is something you both wish to avoid, it's better to discuss the topic openly so you can work together to ensure it doesn't happen.

REASON 2: *'I was afraid she might have taken the question as an insult.'*
This refers to scenarios where you may not have known your partner very long. I suppose I'd have to wonder why you think

someone would take this as an insult. What's wrong with a girl being proactive in this area? What's wrong with a girl being on the Pill, for example? Using contraception is a clear sign she wants to avoid an unplanned pregnancy, which is perfectly valid.

In fact, it shows a lot of responsibility and common sense for a sexually active female to take precautionary measures like this if she feels it is the right decision for her. You should never be afraid to ask this question, because if you're in a sexual relationship with her – even if it's only brief – you should really want to know the answer.

REASON 3: *'I assumed because she didn't mention a condom, she was obviously on the Pill.'*
Don't ever assume this. The stakes are too high so you need to know for sure. As we will discuss in the chapter on consent, don't assume you fully understand what is going on in your partner's mind just because they're not saying anything. She may or may not be on the Pill, or some other method of contraception, but it's too risky to have sex with her first without knowing for sure. The consequences are life-changing if you get this one wrong.

As you're well aware by now, even if she is taking measures to avoid pregnancy, you won't be protected from contracting an STI if you don't use a condom. So, even if condoms aren't mentioned by your partner, you still should use one. Even if she is using contraception, you should still use one. **To be really clear here, unless you're hoping to be a parent and you don't care about contracting an STI, you should always use a condom when you have sex.**

REASON 4: *'I thought it would ruin the moment.'*

Just like some people are reluctant to mention condoms, some lads worry that bringing up contraception would interrupt the flow of things too much. They think it's better to say nothing and just take their chances, silently hoping their partner is taking some measures to prevent a pregnancy.

All of us, girls included, can get totally carried away in a moment. We can become so focused on what's happening in front of us that we're unable to think about the future or the possible consequences of what we're about to do. That's why it's so important to have these conversations early – whether that's asking about condoms or the Pill or any other form of contraception – so that when you and your partner are both aroused and excited you can just enjoy the experience together, knowing you're both protected from the risks of unwanted consequences.

REASON 5: *'I didn't want to ask in case she wasn't using anything and then we'd have to stop.'*

First of all, this only applies to scenarios where you don't have a condom with you, so just have a condom with you and situations like this will never come up. However, if you don't have a condom, and the girl isn't using any contraception, you'd both be taking the maximum level of risk if you went on to have sex with one another. While you may not want to stop, particularly if you're aroused and excited and fully in the moment, this is exactly the kind of scenario you should avoid.

You should make sure that either of you can 'stop' if you're not comfortable, and in all scenarios it's so important you both know how protected you both are. Always ask each other so you know where you stand!

Not asking your male partner to use a condom
REASON 1: *'I didn't want to offend him.'*
Pregnancy is obviously not a concern when two men get together, so all conversations about condom use are aimed at avoiding the spread of STIs. So asking a partner to wear a condom is clearly about protecting you both from catching an infection during sex. Fear of offending him shouldn't be a consideration here, because he should be aware of the risks involved in having unprotected sex.

There's nothing upsetting about wanting you both to be protected, so don't let fear of offending him be the reason you stay quiet on this one. Always bring it up!

REASON 2: *'I knew he'd say no.'*
If any partner of yours is genuinely dead against using a condom, he should be considered a particularly high risk to your sexual health. He is making it pretty clear that unprotected sex is his norm, which significantly increases the likelihood of him picking up and spreading STIs. He obviously doesn't care much for the sexual health of his partners, which should be a concern, especially if you plan to continue in a sexual relationship with him.

REASON 3: *'I was worried it would spoil the moment.'*
Telling your partner to use a condom only takes a second and

could save you both from considerable hassle down the road. It really won't spoil anything, but if that's your concern, just have the conversation long before you get to the bedroom, so it won't interrupt the moment anyway.

Here's another way to look at it – if you think a chat about condom use might spoil things in some way, just imagine how a chat about genital warts or gonorrhoea might go afterwards instead.

REASON 4: *'I was too drunk to care!'*
This is very common, especially among young people. The unavoidable impact of drinking a load of alcohol is that you'll begin to be less concerned about, or aware of, the consequences of your own behaviour. It's why people only get embarrassed about some of their drunken actions the following day as opposed to when they're actually doing them .

This is one area that comes with potentially life-changing consequences, so take extra care to protect yourself at all times. Being 'too drunk to care' is a high-risk and potentially dangerous way for a young person to be in any scenario, especially this one.

REASON 5: *'Neither of us had any symptoms so a condom wasn't needed.'*
Some STIs are symptom-free, which means there are no noticeable signs at all that you may be infected. Either of you could have an STI without realising it, so unprotected sex is not something you should consider. It's so important you know this. Unless you have recently had a sexual health screening neither of you will

know for sure. And don't automatically assume everyone you meet is always telling you the full truth on this one. Even if someone tells you they recently got a screening and were perfectly healthy – ask him to wear one!

Like everything else in this book, this is advice you can take or leave. You are free to make whatever decisions you like here as long as your partner agrees. If having sex without condoms is something you both prefer, then you needn't worry about remembering most of this section. If you prefer not to take on board the info about protection, you'll realise treatments for STIs can be very effective these days. For those of you who wish to find out more information about what it will be like to catch or treat various STIs, check out the appendix at the back of the book for more information.

PREGNANCY

I've spent much of this chapter explaining how to avoid an unplanned pregnancy, but obviously, there may come a time in your life when pregnancy is just what you and your partner want to achieve. **It might seem a long way off to some of you, but there are certain issues to be aware of when you're planning on becoming pregnant.** Let's take a look at some of them now.

Becoming pregnant

I assume you know that a man and a woman need to have sex, first of all, for a pregnancy to occur naturally (if you didn't know this, perhaps this book might be a little advanced for you!). I assume you also realise that for this to happen, all methods of protection and contraception they may have been using previously should be discarded. However, not everyone is aware that timing can also be a key factor when it comes to getting pregnant. There is a specific time during a woman's menstrual cycle when she is most fertile, which is when couples are advised to have regular unprotected sex if pregnancy is the aim. This is why it is so beneficial for a woman to be familiar with her own body and the rhythm of her menstrual cycle so that she knows when she is likely to be ovulating. For women and couples who wish to get pregnant, there is a lot of advice on lifestyle, dietary, exercise and health matters that can help to boost the chances of making it happen.

Miscarriages

Early loss of pregnancies – typically referred to as miscarriages – are very common. Roughly speaking, about one in five pregnancies end in this way. While they can happen for many different reasons, most miscarriages occur in the first 12 weeks of the pregnancy. This is why many expecting parents tend not to tell too many people about their pregnancy until they have reached this point. Miscarriages do occur after the 12-week mark, but they are less common.

In the past, people tended not to discuss their own experiences of miscarriage. It is still an uncomfortable and upsetting topic for people to discuss, but there has been a noticeable increase in recent years in people sharing their experiences in blogs, media interviews and social media posts. We're starting to realise that sharing these experiences with others can help to reduce the stigma associated with miscarriages, while providing support and a sense of community to those who have had this experience.

Reproductive health

If you're like most teenagers, you may think that getting pregnant is something that will automatically happen when you decide the time is right. You might assume you'll just need to stop taking precautions and it will happen for you and your partner straight away. The reality for many people, however, is very different. It can take several years for some couples to become pregnant naturally.

Just like you can get your sexual health tested, you can also monitor your reproductive health throughout adulthood. Tests are available to measure the quality and motility (the ability of sperm to swim the right way) of sperm in men, and the quality and number of eggs in women, for example. Several other tests are available to measure a person's reproductive health or to establish the likelihood of a couple getting pregnant naturally. Some couples may need fertility treatment in order to become pregnant, but there are a wide range of options to those in this position.

Just like miscarriages, however, this can be a very personal area for a lot of people, so it's not something that every couple will decide to speak openly about. However, people are starting to realise how beneficial and supportive it can be to talk honestly with loved ones or with others who have experience of these issues.

Terminations

Prior to the referendum to repeal the 8th Amendment of the Constitution in 2018, it was illegal to terminate a pregnancy in Ireland unless the life of the mother was at risk. Now, terminations, or abortions as they're often referred to, are legally available in Ireland during the first 12 weeks of a pregnancy. This can involve taking medication or undergoing a minor surgical procedure. Abortions are available after the initial 12 weeks of pregnancy only if continuing with the pregnancy puts the mother's life or health at serious risk, or if there is a problem with the development of the foetus which is likely to lead to its death either before or within 28 days of birth.

Abortion can often be a very distressing experience for women and couples to go through, which is why it is widely recommended that people avail of support if they are in this position. This can involve discussions with GPs and staff at family planning clinics as well as availing of supports from mental health professionals, such as therapists and counsellors.

Lessons from the therapy room

Toby

Toby was in his Leaving Cert year when his parents brought him to see me. His girlfriend, Louise, was five months pregnant. His parents were still furious with him for not being more careful and they thought Toby was too immature to become a dad. I think they wanted me to magically turn him into a 30-year-old man overnight so that he'd know how to meet his new responsibilities.

Toby (and Louise) genuinely thought that 'pulling out' before ejaculation – without wearing a condom – was always enough to avoid an unplanned pregnancy. They didn't think condoms were needed to protect them from STIs because neither of them had had previous sexual partners.

Up until that point, there were no conversations in the family about sex, relationships, protection or contraception. His parents felt too awkward to bring up these topics with Toby, even though they knew he was seeing Louise, and Toby was too always too shy to bring it up with them. Even during our sessions, they were all noticeably uncomfortable and reluctant to discuss these topics. His parents hadn't fully appreciated that teenagers need lots of guidance in this area, and Toby wasn't aware how wrong he was in some of his opinions on how to avoid pregnancy.

They wished they hadn't learned the lesson in this way, but they realised young people need to learn about safer sex *before* they are ready to have sex.

Stephen

Stephen was 18 when his mum brought him to see me. His father had died the previous year and she thought it would be a good idea for him to speak to me about how he was feeling. We discussed this issue a lot, and we often spoke about other parts of his life, but after a while I got the feeling that something was bothering him that even his mum didn't know about.

True enough, he told me he was worried about 'weird-coloured discharge' coming from his penis, and for the previous three months it had been sore to urinate. He said he didn't know what to do. He had had unprotected sex while on holiday with mates in Magaluf after the Leaving Cert. He was too afraid to say it to them because he knew they would slag him about it. He didn't want to be known as the guy with an STI like the older brother of one of his mates was (coincidentally, that had also happened in Magaluf, two years earlier). He figured he couldn't tell his mum because he thought she'd be disappointed in him. He didn't want to go to the family GP because the doctor was a family friend and he thought she would tell his mum. And worst of all, as far as he was concerned, he didn't think he could get with anyone again because he thought any girl would dump him and tell her friends once she found out the truth. He felt his life was on hold until this was sorted. The problem was he had no idea how to sort it.

Once he got over the original awkwardness of talking about this problem, we were able to comfortably talk about the solution. Once he realised the GP is forbidden from repeating this to anyone (particularly now that he was 18) and that she'd probably treated hundreds of patients with this condition before, he decided to book an appointment and get his problem treated. Even though he felt uncomfortable having his GP examine his penis, and he certainly didn't enjoy having a syringe inserted into the eye of his penis as part of the process, his symptoms eventually disappeared.

While it's understandable to feel awkward about topics like this, it doesn't do any good to stay quiet about it and avoid getting treatment.

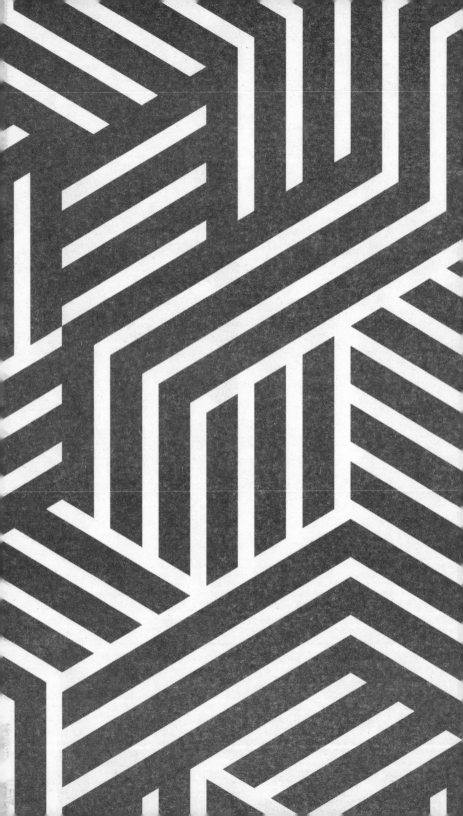

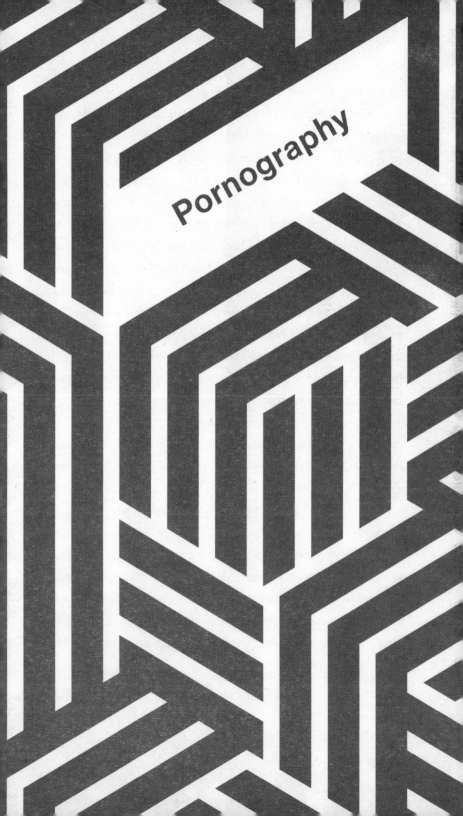

Pornography

If you saw a movie where the main character jumped out of a window and was able to fly to safety because a huge pair of wings appeared magically from his arse, you probably wouldn't mimic the scene the next time you were close to a window, would you? (Well, I hope you wouldn't, anyway!) You'd realise the whole thing was pretty unrealistic, and that it wasn't a fair reflection of how most adults behave when they're next to windows. In fact, you'd probably be able to predict what would happen if you even attempted to do this. Regardless of how things went for the character in the film, you'd know that wings don't magically appear out of people's arses to help them fly out of buildings and that you'd be bang in trouble if you tried it yourself. In other words, when it comes to behaviour like jumping out of buildings with the hope you'll fly to safety, you've enough life experience to tell the difference between fiction and reality.

There's a reason I'm beginning this chapter with a pretty ridiculous example like this. In porn scenes, actors perform in lots of ways, many of which are similar to how most people would behave when they're being intimate with partners. However, there is an increasing amount of material produced by the porn industry showing behaviour that would get you into huge trouble if you mimicked it in real life. The problem is, since most adults shy away from discussing porn with young people, young people don't get any assistance in working out reality from fiction. This chapter, among other things, will help you to be able to spot the difference for yourself.

I'm not here to warn you off watching porn, and I certainly won't try to make you feel embarrassed or ashamed if you enjoy watching people have sex. You're at a stage where it's perfectly normal to be curious and excited about sex and sexuality, so it's pretty reasonable to assume you're at least occasionally interested in seeing naked bodies and scenes of a sexual nature. The purpose of this section is to give you the kind of information that will help you to have healthier experiences when the time comes to have sex yourself, and to help prevent you and your partners from behaving in ways that could harm you both.

Me and porn

I don't remember exactly what age I was when I first saw pornographic material, but it either came in the form of photos in a magazine or footage on a video. I'd say I was either 11 or 12. It's possible that neither you nor any of your friends have ever even seen a porno mag or watched a video (of any kind!), but that's all that was available back then (I'm fully aware this makes me seem ancient!). We didn't have the internet, nor did any of us have access to mobile phones that provided unlimited access to porn sites like nowadays, so there was a lot more work involved than just looking at your mobile if you wanted to see porn as a teenager in the 1990s.

The best you could hope for was that one of your mates got hold of a video. Even if that happened, the problem then was getting access to a video player. Back then, everyone's video players were in the main sitting room by the television (most houses only had one TV, imagine!) so you needed an empty house before you could watch it. And even if you managed that, you were in the company of your mates when it was switched on, a scenario that can obviously start to feel awkward very quickly.

Although 16-year-old me would probably disagree, I'm glad I didn't have as much access to porn back then as you do today, because I got to learn about sex and how to behave with partners from real-life experiences rather than from watching far-fetched scenes from the porn industry that are totally unrealistic.

Let's *not* talk about porn

I don't remember having any conversations about pornography when I was a teenager. Not with any adults, anyway. Teachers didn't once refer to it in any class. There were no mentions of it in my household, and I honestly can't remember seeing the word written in any school textbooks. Back then, pornography just wasn't discussed with teenagers. It was like everyone just pretended it didn't exist.

There were probably lots of reasons people didn't discuss it with young people. First of all, it isn't just you teenagers who often find these conversations awkward and embarrassing – many adults do too. Lots of teachers would find it tricky to have classroom discussions with a room of students about the positives and negatives of porn. Also, many parents might have been unaware their teenagers were even interested in porn, let alone actually watching it. Remember, this is generally not the kind of topic people chat about openly together as a family over breakfast.

Regardless of the reasons, I don't think it's good enough anymore to just avoid these topics because they're awkward. Standing back and letting you or your mates learn about sex and relationships by watching porn is a pretty dismal strategy. While many porn websites show scenes that are realistic and healthy, plenty of sites show behaviour that is harmful and unhealthy, giving young people misguided expectations of how most people enjoy sex in the real world.

THE WORLD ACCORDING TO PORN

In the world of porn, every social interaction leads to sex, obviously. If someone makes eye contact with you, they want you. If you're on a bus, someone sitting close by wants to have sex with you right away. If you're in a taxi, keep in mind that the driver is always up for it. If you're falling short on your college grades, your lecturer will most likely want to have sex with you as a punishment. If you have a stepsibling, they fantasise about you constantly. If you have a stepparent, they're just waiting for the opportunity to sleep with you too. Sex is an acceptable means of payment to every landlord if you're short on cash. If you get a job as an electrician, plumber, pool attendant or takeaway driver, for example, you can expect every customer to answer the door half-naked with the intention of having sex with you. Actually, if you even get an interview for a job, you can bank on having sex with the person interviewing you before it finishes. In fact, if you have any kind of interaction with someone and it *doesn't* lead to sex, there must be something wrong with you.

All girls are keen for their best friends to join in every time they have sex. They rarely wear underwear because you don't need underwear when all you do is have sex. Your girlfriend will definitely be OK with your friends watching you both have sex. Also, she'd prefer if you shouted really demeaning things at her during sex. The more you call her a slut and a whore, for example, the more she'll know you like her. Actually, she'll think more of you the ruder and more abusive you become. Nobody wears condoms. Everyone likes threesomes and group sex. There's no reason to learn about consent because you're meant to ignore the word 'no' if you ever hear it in the bedroom. Come to think of it, I don't know why I said 'bedroom' there, because people are equally keen to have sex in whatever location they happen to be as soon as you meet them. Even if someone says 'no' they secretly mean 'yes'. This is particularly true of anyone drunk, and *all* women. Nobody remains faithful in relationships. Weirdly, this is especially true on people's wedding nights. If you're short of money anywhere, if you're lost or if you need any kind of assistance, the answer is always to have sex with someone nearby. That'll get you out of trouble.

In summary, every move you make should lead you to having sex as soon as possible.

IT'S NOT
GOOD
ENOUGH
TO AVOID
THESE
TOPICS
BECAUSE
THEY'RE
AWKWARD.

All lads have massive penises, and they all come every time they have sex. Even if they're in a room with several naked women at the same time – which happens everyone pretty regularly, remember – every single one of their partners will be having the time of their lives. All women reach orgasm every time you touch them, and no man has ever struggled to get or keep an erection. Every sexual experience is unbelievably satisfying for everyone involved and nobody is even remotely self-conscious about their own body. In fact, the sad truth about life is that the days just aren't long enough for us all to be having the amount of sex that we secretly want.

IMPORTANT FACT:
If even one sentence on the previous pages seems
reasonable to you, you're watching way too much porn!

THE POSITIVES OF PORN

This may be the first time you've ever read about the positives of porn. After all, it's not a topic people spend much time writing about, particularly in books written for lads your age. Most people prefer to warn young people about the negatives of porn and leave it at that, but that would leave out a big and important chunk of the conversation. **Like a lot of things in life, there are good and bad elements to porn, so it's important to acknowledge that and discuss what they are.**

Porn has a massive global audience of people your age and older. In fact, in the workshops I've done with lads about porn, most people said they first saw porn between the ages of 11 and 13.

Some were younger, others were slightly older, but the majority first saw porn footage when they were still children. And just so you know, the appeal of porn doesn't go away automatically just because you get older. Individuals and couples of all ages consume porn in lots of different ways throughout their adult lives. Some have no interest in it, others are disgusted by it, while plenty of people around the world have never seen it. Obviously, porn can also be very harmful for people who work in the industry and for people who view the material (we'll get to that shortly!), but this section is about why young people can find it a positive.

Lads are usually surprised when I ask them about the positives of watching porn, but once they start to consider their answers, they usually have a lot to say. Here are some of the most common replies I get from 16-year-olds when I ask about the benefits of watching porn.

'We learn about sex.'

I hear this answer more than any other, and it's very easy to understand why. Since chats about sex are often really awkward for adults and young people, and young people don't have any real-life experiences yet themselves, porn is often their main outlet for learning about sex. For some people, seeing porn was their earliest lesson in their sex education. It was the first time they realised 'what goes where' when two people are having sex. Most people are fairly horrified by the messiness of the whole thing when they see it first, particularly if they're very young. But during adolescence, it's pretty normal to be curious and aroused by sex scenes, so porn can become a go-to place for learning about loads of other aspects of sex and intimacy.

'We learn the different positions.'

Porn is the only place you'll see actual demonstrations of what sex can be like, but pretty quickly, you'll realise there are many different ways for people to enjoy the experience. There are lots of different sex positions, all of which are recreated throughout the porn industry for viewers to enjoy. Adults have their own experiences to refer to, but young people generally don't, which makes porn footage their primary source of info for this area too. After all, not everyone would be mad about the prospect of discussing sex positions with a parent or a teacher, so porn takes their place as the educator.

'We can learn different techniques.'

It's very understandable to want to do something 'right' when you try it for the first time. Whether it's driving, skiing, kissing or having sex, most people agree it's better to know what you're doing than to be totally clueless. It's one thing knowing *what* to do, but it's also important to know *how* to do it. That's why many lads say that porn is a useful source of examples and demonstrations of how to do everything from kissing to sex and everything in between, so that when they have their own experience they'll feel more competent and better prepared for things to go well.

'It teaches you about foreplay.'

Sexual activity involves way more than just intercourse, remember. You should know by now that for intercourse to occur, the penis needs to be erect. If you're having sex with a girl, the vagina also needs to be moist or else it could be incredibly painful for your partner (and also for you). Foreplay can help with both of these aims. The range of ways a couple can achieve both of these things during foreplay is both vast and really enjoyable. Everything from cuddling and kissing to oral sex and mutual masturbation is included in the list of ways people arouse themselves and each other. Sometimes these activities lead to sex, but often they don't. As we covered in the chapter on safer sex, there are many different ways for you and your partner to please yourselves and each other *without* having penetrative sex. Remember, foreplay gives you all the fun but fewer of the risks that come with having sex, such as unwanted pregnancy. Either way, porn can be a rich source of information and guidance for young people in this area.

'It helps you to work out what you like.'

Like any group of people who haven't experienced something for themselves, not all young people know what they'd be comfortable doing with their future partners. For many, it can just be trial and error until they find something they really enjoy. Some people, however, can get an indication of what they'd like from watching porn scenes. They get a sense of what they'd like to experience with partners, and just as importantly, they also realise what they'd be uncomfortable or unwilling to try. The key thing to remember here is that people have their own tastes and desires. You have your own boundaries and your partners will have theirs, and it's really important you both understand what they are. Once you get that part right, your job then is to discuss and agree with one another what you'd be comfortable doing together. We don't all like the same things, and porn can be a useful guide to help people discover what would work for them.

'It helps you to work out your sexual orientation if you weren't sure.'

This is similar to the last answer. Since people usually watch porn in privacy, they can search for footage they most want to watch. Many people have no questions around their own sexuality, meaning they have a clear idea whether they'd like relationships with men or women, both, or neither. They don't have any doubts. But lots of people spend their teenage years – and often much of their adult lives – trying to work this out. They question their sexuality in their own minds. Some people are comfortable to talk openly about their uncertainty; others prefer to keep it to themselves. Either way, porn can provide some people with the space and privacy to explore this question themselves.

'It helps you to know what women want you to do, because obviously we don't have a clue yet.'

This is a common answer, and a bit of a controversial one too. First of all, it's perfectly normal to assume that if you keep seeing female porn performers respond in a particular way to certain behaviour, you'll get a good idea of how women in real life would respond to the same thing. However, this is somehow both an understandable way to think *and* a really dangerous way to think, and I'll explain why. It's a common-sense way to think, for obvious reasons. After all, if you're keen to learn what would please your partner, basing your assumptions on what pleases the only group of women you've ever seen have sex – female porn performers – makes complete sense. However, and this is where things become a little trickier, what if the women in the scenes aren't enjoying it, and they're only acting as if they are because it's their job to convince everyone watching that they're having a great time? This might be a fairly harmless issue if they were only pretending to have orgasms, for example, or pretending to be really enjoying themselves when they're not, but it gets a lot more serious if they act as if they, say, love being hit during sex when they actually don't. What if they act as if they love being spat on or shouted at aggressively? What if they act as if they love being physically hurt? The danger in scenes like these is that they give inexperienced people (which is everyone around your age) the impression that not only is it OK to hit or physically hurt women during sex, but that they actually like it. Remember the silly example I gave at the start of this chapter about the dangers of jumping out of windows expecting to fly to safety just because you've seen it in a movie? This is exactly the kind of thing I was thinking of when I wrote that. Women being physically mistreated or verbally abused during sex is not the kind of behaviour you should re-enact in real life just because you've seen it in a porn scene. It is completely wrong to assume sex should automatically include this behaviour. In fact, hitting women – or men – or physically hurting them in any way is illegal.

The reality is that the majority of porn is made with a male audience in mind, and it portrays girls and women as mere objects for male satisfaction. The message is that these sex objects may be treated in any way a man wishes, and what's more, the female will not only enjoy it, but will be turned on by it. This is an absurd myth that boys your age are having great difficulty with. Many young men are finding out the hard way that some of the lessons they learned from porn have sent them down the wrong path in their sex lives. This leads us nicely into the next section of this chapter, which is all about some of the things you need to learn about sex which porn *won't* teach you ...

THE STUFF YOU WON'T LEARN FROM WATCHING PORN

The importance of consent

You'll learn a lot about consent from reading the 'Consent' chapter in this book. However, if porn was your only teacher when it comes to sex and relationships, you'd know very little about consent. As I'll explain in that chapter, consent is all about communication and respect. In the real world, the ideal scenario is that a couple are comfortable enough to let each other know how they are feeling about whatever activity they are doing together – whether that's walking in the park or having sex in a bed – and they both respond respectfully to what each other says. In a nutshell, if one of you wants to stop, change or take a break from what you're doing, it's perfectly reasonable to assume you won't be forced to continue against your will. It's pretty straightforward when you think about it.

In the world of porn, however, you'll get a lot of mixed messages on this. There are loads of scenarios where performers respond respectfully and enthusiastically to what their partner wants, but – and this is the crucially important part – you are very likely to come across footage where this doesn't happen at all. Scenes where people's objections are ignored are common. Footage of people being forced to do things against their will is common. Scenarios where people forcefully do things to others are common. Scenes where people are mistreated, manhandled, groped, abused, assaulted and raped are all over the internet. They are so common and widely available that you could be forgiven for thinking this is perfectly acceptable behaviour. And in the vast majority of scenes, the people being mistreated are women. If you didn't have anyone telling you otherwise, you might think this is how *you* should behave towards women. You might think it's acceptable to ignore them or overrule them if they say they don't want to do what you want to do, because that's what happens in porn!

This message won't appear on screen at the end of the footage, but it's important you know that these aren't scenes of consensual sexual activity; they're scenes showing crimes taking place. This is why porn is such a poor teacher when it comes to consent.

How to protect yourself

You've learned plenty about contraception from reading the previous chapter, but you'll learn next to nothing about it if your only source of information is porn. Obviously, it's worth saying that not all porn scenes follow the same plotlines or scripts. There's a huge variety in locations, dialogue, scenes and plots, as well as levels of acting and entertainment. Pretty much every sexual activity appears on screen somewhere in the porn industry, but you'll rarely ever see responsible discussions about the importance of protection against STIs and unwanted pregnancies. You tend not to see couples patiently chatting about which methods of contraception would suit them best. In some scenes, you may see men using condoms, but discussions about the reasons for doing so are rarely included in the final edit of the film. **If porn was your only source of info on sex and relationships, we'd totally understand if you didn't even know what a condom was, let alone why you would use one.** We'd understand why you didn't have a clue about methods of birth control that women could use. And most worrying of all, we'd totally get why you'd spend a great deal of your adult life having sexually transmitted diseases and dealing with crisis pregnancies. So be wary of assuming what you see in porn is everything you need to know!

What's monogamy?!

Most people would be uncomfortable knowing their partner was having lots of sex with other people behind their back, but in porn, that's what everyone seems to be doing. In the world of porn, nobody turns down the chance for sex because they are committed to someone else. Everyone is up for it all the time, and even on their own wedding nights they're willing to cheat on their partners. If porn was your go-to for guidance on this one, you'd laugh off the idea of ever being faithful to your partner. In the real world, though, being faithful to one another is an essential part of the vast majority of relationships.

It's important you don't think I'm saying that cheating doesn't happen in real life. It happens a lot! What I'm saying is that porn doesn't give many examples of people being faithful. You won't see many scenes where people turn down sex because they're honouring the commitments they made to their partners. It's as if that kind of behaviour doesn't exist at all. Obviously, it's up to you how you behave when you're in a relationship yourself, but don't base your behaviour solely on what you've seen in porn.

In fact, quite a lot of porn depicts a way of life that isn't as close to balanced reality as you may think. In the same way that being unable to say no to a drink would be considered a problem, being infatuated with sex and constantly being on the lookout for opportunities to have sex are a cause for concern. In both cases, it is likely that the person has become addicted. The world of porn presents this as the way to live your best life, but the reality is often very different.

It's not all about you!

Every single porn scene is different. Even if the set-up/script is similar from scene to scene, the behaviour of the actors will be different, and the levels of pleasure experienced by each of them will vary. **A fundamental part of any sexual encounter – from a kiss to having sex – is that the people involved are not only consenting, but are also experiencing pleasure.** However, if your only knowledge of what sex entails comes from porn, and you only watched scenes between men and women, you'd be forgiven for thinking sex is about one thing – getting the man to ejaculate! In porn, most of the behaviour (actions and words) is aimed at this outcome. There is often very little time spent ensuring the female is experiencing pleasure too. However, in real life, ensuring that both you and your partner are enjoying your-selves is a fundamental part of the experience. So, whether your partners are male or female, approaching every encounter as an opportunity for you both to experience pleasure is the healthiest approach. You may not get that impression if porn is all you know!

It's OK not to be in the mood

If you relied on porn to teach you, you'd be forgiven for thinking there is no scenario in the real world where at least one person in the room doesn't want to have sex immediately. Everyone's at it! Pizza delivery guys, plumbers, swimming pool cleaners, gar-deners, college lecturers, taxi drivers – every single time they go to work they end up having sex! This may or may not come as a total surprise to you, but this is nothing like the real world. It's true to say that sometimes people can act on impulse, and that spontaneous sexual encounters occur. In fact, many people use dating apps specifically for this reason. However, if you thought the porn industry was a reflection of how everyone lives, you'd find yourself having to awkwardly apologise very often for making inappropriate advances towards everyone you meet! The reality is, everyone – both men and women – have different levels of arousal and interest in having sex. We're all different, and we all have days where we're not interested in being intimate with other people. This is perfectly normal; it's just that you'd never think it was if you relied only on porn to learn about adult behaviour.

We're all different shapes and sizes

If you went through the list of most popular male porn actors and performers, you'd see they have very similar body shapes. They're generally fairly ripped – six-packs, toned muscles, low body fat – and all have larger-than-average penises. It's worth knowing that many of their bodies have been surgically enhanced to look a certain way (yes, even their penises!) so be wary of assuming this is what all men's bodies are meant to look like. The same applies to the appearance of female performers. If you base your expectations of real-life partners on what you see in porn, you're in for a big surprise. Surgically enhanced boobs and shaved vulvas are commonplace in porn, but that's not a true representation of what you will encounter in the real world with women from your own community. People are well aware how damaging places like Instagram can be for their self-esteem and body image – where people constantly compare themselves negatively to others – but porn can warp your thinking around what you and your partners are meant to look like. **It's a big mistake to base your expectations of men's and women's bodies on what you see most often in porn films.** We're all different shapes and sizes, remember. Regardless of what shape you are or how you feel about your own body, relying on porn to guide you in this area isn't the healthiest approach.

Sex talk

In some scenes, it's easy to tell the dialogue between the performers is scripted. During the 'sex talk', if you listen to it, the female is often being spoken to as a sex object. Not every scene is like this, obviously, but there can be lots of aggressive, objectifying, abusive and demeaning language towards women in porn films. Every couple is different, and every person has their own idea of what they are comfortable with, but don't assume it is appropriate to speak to female partners in real life in the same way you've heard them spoken to in films. In many cases, speaking to them in the crude, insulting ways you may have seen in porn films will put an end to the sexual encounter. In fact, verbally abusing your partner during sex may bring an end to the relationship altogether. Be warned!

Aggression

Following on from the point about abusive and insulting vocabulary, depictions of aggression and violence towards women are common in porn. Years ago, scenes in which women were mistreated were restricted to the edges of the industry, but they're very much a part of mainstream porn now. Be careful not to lazily assume that every behaviour in a porn film is an example of how you should behave when you are old enough to have sex yourself. As you would with every other film you watch, develop the capacity to critically reflect on the content. (We're back to the jumping out of windows thing again!) **Don't assume women enjoy being physically mistreated because you saw a porn film in which this happened.**

It is appropriate and normal for lads your age to be curious about sex, so it shouldn't be a source of shame or embarrassment if you are. It's common sense to think you'll learn about sex by watching sex, so there's no need to be self-critical if you've allowed porn to shape your expectations on what sex entails. It's understandable also that you'd want to know as much as possible before your first experience of sex or sexual activity. Watching porn can be an easier, less embarrassing way to find out about sex than asking parents, older siblings, teachers or friends, for example, but that doesn't mean it's the right place to go for information and guidance. You know by now that, while porn can be pleasurable and exciting to watch, it can be a very one-dimensional and damaging way to learn about sex.

Like everyone else, you get to decide for yourself what kind of relationship you have with porn. You might ignore it, watch it occasionally or watch it a lot. You might be sickened by it or excited by it. Whatever your approach to porn or your attitude towards watching it, please remember that wings won't appear from your arse if you try to fly out a window!

THE REAL WORLD VS THE PORN WORLD

If you haven't realised by now, there's a pretty substantial difference between the porn industry and the real world when it comes to attitudes to sex and sexual behaviour. See if you can guess which of the two possible outcomes in each of the following scenarios is more likely to happen in real life or in porn.

Trevor

Trevor tells his girlfriend, Claire, that he really fancies her best friend, Shauna. He says he thinks Shauna is unbelievably sexy and that he has always had a thing for her. He then spends a few more minutes explaining what he likes about Shauna's appearance, especially her body.

1. To show how much she loves Trevor, Claire blindfolds him and organises a threesome with Shauna as a birthday present. This goes so well it becomes a regular thing.

2. Claire ends the relationship with Trevor immediately. She tells Shauna what he said, and they both agree he's a pig who should be avoided. When word gets out among their friends, he becomes known as 'Threesome Trev' to everyone and is slagged about it for years after. He now says it's the biggest mistake of his life.

Graham

Graham, an engineering lecturer, offers to stay back after class to help Louise, one of his students, with her assignment. During the course of their chat, he starts to rub her back suggestively and says something very crude about her body. Unknown to Graham, Louise has been recording the conversation, so she won't forget any important advice he gives her.

1. Louise quickly leaves the room and reports him to the university authorities straight away. Graham is immediately suspended pending an investigation into her allegation. He is eventually sacked, and his wife leaves him. He can't get a job again anywhere because details of this case appeared in the media.

2. Louise giggles and says this is what she's been waiting her whole college life to hear, and they have passionate sex. It's one of the best days Graham has ever had at work.

Alice and Mary-Kate

Alice and Mary-Kate are 19-year-old twin sisters. They both fancy their middle-aged neighbour Gavin, so they decide to sneak into his home with the hope of seducing him together while his wife is asleep.

1. Gavin rings the police, and they are both arrested for breaking into his property. Gavin and his wife immediately tell the girls' parents what happened. Details of the incident later appear on social media for everyone in their family, college and neighbourhood to see. The girls are so mortified they can't leave their house again for months.

2. Gavin says he was expecting their arrival, invites them inside and they all have sex with one another. Gavin's wife hears them and gets up to join in. It all goes so well it becomes a regular thing for them all.

Brian

Brian really fancies his stepsister, Fiona, who has recently moved into his home with her mum. One night when his dad and Fiona's mum are out of the house, he decides to go to her bedroom in the hope of seeing her undress. She catches him at the door while she is half-naked.

1. Fiona is initially shocked to see him, but despite being half-naked, sparks up a conversation with him about feeling lonely in her new surroundings. She invites him to sit on the bed to chat further, suggesting that sex would be a

great way for her to feel more at home. Every one of Brian's fantasies comes true.

2. Fiona screams when she sees him and then rings her mum. Brian runs back to his bedroom, full of regret and knowing he's in huge trouble. Since he can't be trusted to respect people's boundaries or privacy, he is kicked out of the house and told to go live with his mum, who lives alone. Everyone in school finds out and he is a laughing stock.

IMPORTANT REMINDER:
Don't rely on the porn industry to help you understand or predict how people will behave. I hope these pretty absurd examples made that point very clearly!

DON'T LET PORN HIJACK YOUR SEXUALITY!

As you can tell by now, I'm not here to lecture you on the dangers of porn or any other aspect of adult living that you may be experiencing for the first time. My aim is to help prepare you for whatever life has in store for you, both now and in the future. Your sexuality is emerging and developing in its own unique way, but it would be wrong if I didn't let you know about a particular problem for young men that I see very regularly in my therapy practice. **Put simply, porn is hijacking the sexuality of lads all over Ireland.** I'm going to explain what I mean by using you as an example.

I'll start by assuming you are someone interested in having relationships with other people (I'm saying that because virtually everyone is like this!). My next assumption isn't true of every young lad in Ireland, but it's true for the majority – you enjoy watching porn, and you're having far more sexual experiences on your own in front of screens than with real people in the real world. Maybe you already know who you're attracted to, maybe you're unsure, but either way, you imagine a future where you have fulfilling sex in healthy relationships with people you really like. For the purposes of this example, I'll assume you like girls. You know there will be good days and bad days in your future relationships, but you're excited by the prospect of having many different experiences that you really enjoy. In other words, you'll be having sex for real with women instead of having it virtually by watching performers in porn. You're very excited by this.

However, I want you to jump to being three years older than you are now. Imagine that your sex life is dominated by watching porn on your own. Your interest in having sex with other people is fading. Having spent the time between now and then using porn as your biggest sexual influence, you believe the following things to be true. The purpose of any and all sexual activity is for you to come. The way you should treat women during sex is to verbally abuse them and, in some cases, act violently towards them. You aren't that interested in women you meet because they look nothing like the ones you see in porn scenes. You can't be bothered committing time and effort into a real relationship because porn can satisfy you instantly whenever you want it to. On the very rare occasions you actually find yourself in a bedroom with a girl, you can't get an erection because this real-life scene is nowhere near as arousing as the fantasy you're used to watching on the internet. If you do find yourself being sexual with a girl, it's likely that your head will be replaying porn scenes. Your body will be present but your mind will be elsewhere, scrolling through your memory bank of porn fantasies. In summary, you've lessened your interest in real-life relationships because porn has taken over your sexuality and is completely in charge. You've now moved into the territory of porn addiction and it's time to find support.

Most lads who find themselves in this situation would have laughed off the suggestion that it would be in their future if I had told them three years earlier. But warnings like this aren't shared with young people because people are still so awkward talking about porn. Hopefully, this made-up example is as close as you'll ever find yourself to being in that situation.

Lessons from the therapy room

Neil

Neil was 19 when his parents brought him to see me. He had recently decided to leave his college course at the end of the first semester in first year and they felt he needed help to decide what he wanted to do next. After a few sessions with just the two of us, Neil and myself started to talk about relationships and how he felt about being with someone. He said he hadn't kissed anyone yet, and he spoke openly about watching porn on a daily basis. I wondered whether he was eager for some real-life experiences, but he laughed off the suggestion. Girls in real life don't look like girls in porn, he said, so he didn't think he should 'lower his standards'. He spoke as if spending time masturbating alone watching online porn was better than anything the real world could offer. He talked about certain porn scenes as if he was a participant in them himself. It was clear he had grown such an unhealthy attachment to 'virtual' sex that he was depriving himself of any opportunity to enjoy the real thing with a real partner. After a few conversations about his relationship to porn and how it was turning him off real-life experiences, Neil started to realise what was happening. He could see how he had been living in a porn 'bubble', far removed from reality, which was setting him up for a life of fantasy and isolation. For a while Neil battled with this – part of him thought what he had been doing was fine, and that it was his own business, but the other part was really concerned about where his life was going. The more he grappled with this, the more motivated he became to return to the world outside of porn and to have experiences with actual people.

Keith

Keith was 18 when his parents brought him to see me. They said he seemed miserable and lonely, which was not like him at all. He wasn't giving them any explanations and they were very concerned, so they brought him to therapy in the hope it would help. They were right to be worried, because Keith was in a bad place. He started to speak about his situation after a few sessions once his parents had left the room. His girlfriend Gigi had broken up with him recently because of his treatment of her during sex. Despite telling him several times that she didn't like it when he held her by the throat, Keith didn't listen. Despite being told several times not to shout insults at her during sex, he didn't change his behaviour. Gigi found it very upsetting that she kept having to tell him and was furious that he wasn't listening. She broke up with him, and all his friends soon found out the reason why. He was gutted it was over because he really liked her, and was really embarrassed. He stayed in his house because he couldn't face the prospect of anyone asking him about it. I figured porn had something to do with this, so we started to speak about it. Keith had been watching porn regularly since he was 12. He had become so familiar with how porn performers shout at partners that he was doing it without realising it. He had become so used to men being aggressive and rough to women in porn that he constantly wanted to do the same. It turned out Keith genuinely didn't know the difference between appropriate sexual behaviour and (illegal) sexual assault. He soon realised that Gigi could have pressed charges against him for how he treated her, but it took a lot longer to undo the negative impact porn was having on his sexual behaviour.

Greg

Greg came to see me on his own when he was 21. After several sessions talking about other issues, he opened up about his relationship with porn, saying that was the main reason he came to therapy in the first place. He was wondering if he was addicted because he watched it so much. He couldn't get an erection with a partner lately and was anxious that all his time watching porn was the cause. Also, he had begun to watch gay porn, saying that he was just 'bored' of seeing the same kinds of scenes over and over with women who all looked the same. He was sure he wasn't gay, a topic we explored at length. He was very confused as to how he had found himself in a position where he seemed more interested in watching sex online than having real-life experiences. Greg was worried he had gone too far into the world of porn to be able to return to reality. I explained to Greg how the adolescent brain works – it's constantly seeking new and novel experiences. On porn sites, the algorithms manipulate this in such a way to keep people consuming more and more porn by enticing them into new and more exciting ways of experiencing virtual sex. He realised that his relationship with porn was preventing him having a sex life that involved other people. Over the course of our work together, Greg committed to gradually changing his behaviour because he was very concerned about his chances of having a proper relationship with a real person in the future. He began by trying to masturbate without watching porn, then trying to watch less porn, then making more of an effort to interact with actual people rather than the fantasy of online performers he would never meet. He was one of many young men who came to see me with this issue. They realised the unhealthy impact porn was having on their sexual development, but thankfully for them all, they had reached the stage where they were willing to do something about it.

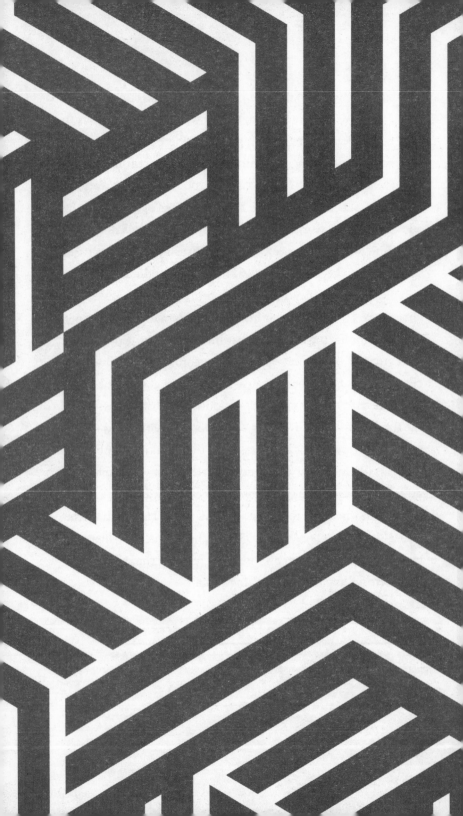

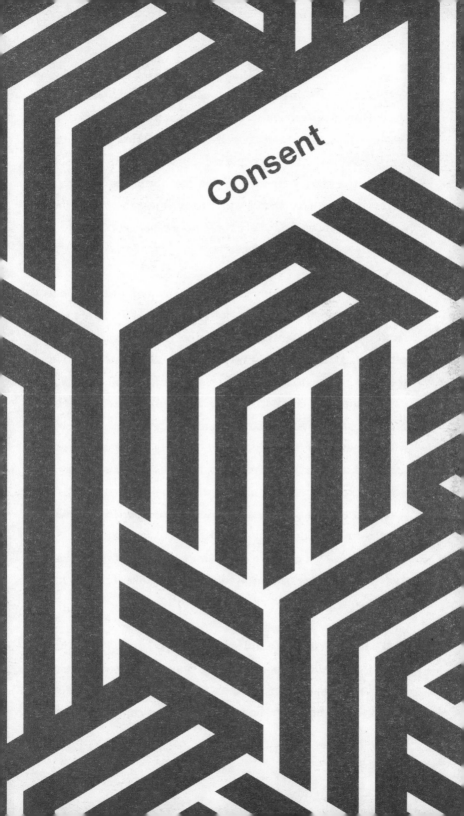

Consent

I'm going to start this chapter by asking some questions. Of all the times you've seen consent mentioned on social media or in the news, how often was it a positive news story? How many times was it a tale about how a couple consented to a really enjoyable and positive sexual experience? Did the story refer to a scene where consent was present or where consent was absent? In other words, was it about the joys of a consensual experience or the pain of a non-consensual experience?

I'm going to guess that if you've seen many news stories about consent on TV or online, the majority of them – if not all of them – were upsetting accounts or allegations of non-consensual sexual activity. Basically, it was always bad news. At least one person in the story experienced pain, distress or trauma, and there was usually someone else portrayed as a villain. Stories about the benefits of consent or the ways people happily consented to being with one another probably haven't come up too often on your feed, if at all. That's because when it comes to sexual consent, positive experiences aren't newsworthy. People tend not to think it's a big deal when people have consensual sex together, or when couples can chat openly about what they're comfortable to do. Therefore, when it comes to discussing consent or developing an understanding of what's involved, you'd be forgiven for thinking it's all about victims and villains.

Well, I'm going to take a different approach here. This section is not going to be all about ensuring you always avoid the roles of victim or villain. Don't get me wrong, I hope you never know what it's like to be either. I hope you never experience pain around consent and that you never hurt anyone else, but reducing the crime rate isn't the focus of this book. **Instead, I'll be discussing ways of ensuring you and your partner know you're both consenting, so that you have better, safer, more enjoyable sexual experiences.**

Me and consent

This is a little difficult to write, and it might be difficult to read, but unfortunately my earliest memories of anything to do with consent are not very pleasant at all. Most conversations about consent, especially when they're with teenage boys, tend to be aimed at ensuring you treat girls respectfully at all times. That seems to be everyone's main focus. Often, however, a big and important piece of the conversation is left out – the part about supporting you to ensure other people treat you and your body respectfully too. When I was a teenager, my body wasn't treated respectfully at all by a physio who I was seeing to help me recover from a football injury. It took me many years to tell people about what happened, but it was obviously a very difficult thing to go through back then. It was something that had a long-lasting impact on me as I grew older, but when I was able to talk about it, supportive people made a real difference. In fact, I couldn't have healed without their help. I'm telling you this because when you read about the importance of respecting people's bodies through-out this chapter, **I want you to keep in mind that you and your body are worthy of the same respect too.** I don't know if reading a book like this would have made me handle that situation any differently back then. I suppose there's no way of knowing something like that. My reason for writing this section is to help you have a better understanding of what consent is all about so that you'll be likely to have more positive experiences as a result.

Let's *not* talk about consent

I have no memories from my teenage years of someone speaking to me about consent. I heard the word 'consent' used often, obviously, but never once in relation to sexual activity. It was usually written on medical forms where I was asked if I consented to various procedures. Maybe lots of other people were having lengthy and detailed conversations with teenagers about this topic, but I never heard them. Back then, as you can probably gather by now, adults didn't do much talking to teenagers about sex at all. **Since we didn't talk about sex, we couldn't hear about consent, so we all grew up without learning anything about it.** A few times during civics class (ask your parents!) the teacher spoke about being respectful to girls in general, which was probably as far as he was willing to go in talking about any kind of sexual activity. (Obviously, he never once considered any of us would be interested in having same-sex relationships!) Avoiding any chat about sexual activity among teenagers is fine if you just want an easy life, but it means you can't give them any guidance or information on this aspect of growing up. I'm going to be taking a very different approach to that throughout this chapter.

WHAT IS CONSENT?

Put simply, consent is present in any sexual encounter when the people involved are willingly participating and fully informed. In other words, when everyone is happy to take part and understands what is happening.

I'll get to some of the trickier questions around this later in the chapter, but the simplest way to ensure you have more fulfilling and positive experiences is to keep two very basic but important things in mind – *respect* and *communication*. In other words, you both talk to one another about how you feel about what is happening, or what you would both like to happen. You always take your partner's wishes into consideration, because sexual activity should always be on both people's terms. If you can get a handle on both of these when you're engaged in sexual activity with one another, you'll both have a much better time together.

IT'S GOOD TO TALK

I'm sure you've heard the phrase 'it's good to talk'. It's often used in mental health campaigns to encourage people to discuss their feelings and thoughts with others. Along the same lines as 'a problem shared is a problem halved', it's a phrase that's used to urge people to talk openly and regularly during times of difficulty. While I strongly agree that it's really helpful to let other people know what's going on in your head (I am a therapist, after all!) – I also think that's a really good way to approach sexual activity. Before I explain what I mean, I'll first explain what I *don't* mean.

I don't mean that we should all start talking really openly about our own sexual experiences. I don't think it's a good idea to throw up a load of details on Snapchat, for example, about what you and your partner enjoy doing together. I don't think it's a good idea to interrupt the next class you have to share those details with the teacher and your classmates. It's probably not wise to blurt out some specifics at the next family lunch either.

When I say people should talk more openly about sex, I'm referring to the times when you're alone with your partner. In those moments, especially when you're being intimate with one another, I believe it's *really* good to talk!

Like I said at the start of this chapter, most stories about consent are about people having bad experiences. Either someone didn't listen to what was being said, or couldn't communicate what they thought, or they just did what they wanted with someone without saying a thing. Rather than focusing on the risks, dangers and implications of non-consensual sexual behaviour, let's look at how you can ensure you and your partner know you're both on the same page when you're together. In other words, how to ensure you're both consenting to whatever you're doing sexually together. And the best way by far to achieve that is by talking.

Consent is about agreement. It's about jointly deciding on doing something together. It doesn't matter what it is, who suggests it, or how it's phrased, consent is achieved if you both agree to do it together. Remember, the simplest and most effective way to let someone know how you feel about something is to tell them. The easiest and most accurate way to know how your partner feels is to ask them. If you and your partner get this bit right, and you can both talk openly about what you enjoy, then you will massively increase your chances of having better experiences. In other words, the more you communicate with one another, the better the sex will be!

Most people your age would be well aware that sex involves far more than the bit where there's penetration, and that there are plenty of times when couples are intimate with one another where it doesn't even involve that. If you were about eleven or twelve years old, I might feel the need to run through the various ways people can be sexual with one another, but you're well past that point. You know by now that couples can have hugely satisfying experiences without any penetration happening. So, sexual consent is all about finding the place that you *both* want to be, and then trying to enjoy the experience as much as possible. However, you'll both make this task a lot trickier to manage if neither of you says a word to one another!

YOU'RE NOT THE BOSS!

Have you ever been told you can't do something you really want to do? I'm going to assume the answer is yes. There's no way you've gotten to this stage of your life without hearing your parents, teachers, friends, neighbours or siblings say the word 'no'. When you were a kid, there were times when you weren't allowed to stay up as late as you wanted. This is a pretty basic example of being told 'no' but it's an experience that virtually everyone has had. I'm sure you've had countless experiences throughout your life when you've asked questions and got answers you didn't like. And since it's totally normal for teenagers to want more freedom than the adults in their lives are willing to give, you're probably also familiar with the word 'no' when it comes to negotiating with your parents around pretty much anything. *Can I stay out another hour? Can I stay home from school? Will you give me more money? Can I go out tonight? Will you buy me new clothes? Can I stay on the Xbox?* ... The list is endless.

It's a familiar pattern – you want things to go one way, but your parents are on a different wavelength. You might do your best to put your point of view across but you have to accept there's certain things you just can't do without their approval. Since this is familiar to virtually every teenager, there's no need for me to go on about this much longer. Basically, you've had to realise – sometimes the hard way – that you're not the one in charge.

Throughout your whole life, in fact, you've gradually realised that an important aspect of growing up is learning to accept and respect boundaries. In other words, you don't get to do something just because you want to do it. While it's often tough to hear this, and it can be hard to accept sometimes, it's crucially important knowledge to bring with you into relationships. And I'm not just talking about times when you're being sexual or intimate with partners.

Before I get to the sex side of things, I'll mention a really obvious example of what I mean. If you want to see a certain film in the cinema, and your partner wants to see something else, you've got some talking to do. Unless you're both happy to go separately and alone to see each film – not everyone's idea of a fun date! – you need to work things out between you. Whatever you end up doing together, it's pretty clear that you both need to agree. It's not reasonable to insist someone sees a film against their will, and it's not fair (or legal!) to force them to see it either. If you can't agree which film to see together, you'll have to go your separate ways or else come up with another plan for the evening ahead.

As I'm sure you're realising, this is all pretty basic common-sense stuff so far. To be honest, it doesn't get much more complicated when it comes to sexual activity (unless alcohol is involved – which I'll get to later). Some people find the issue of consent really difficult to grasp, but if you can get your head round the example with the cinema, you'll have no issue with this. In basic terms – consent is about expressing what you both would like to do, and coming to an agreement on what to do together. And remember, if it's not OK for one of you, it's not OK. After that, it's up to you both to try to make it as enjoyable as possible for yourselves and each other.

THE AGE OF CONSENT

If you didn't already know, the age of consent in Ireland is 17. This is the legal age at which people are seen as mature enough to consent to sex. If someone older than 17 is sexually involved with someone below that age, a law has been broken. Now, you might turn around and ask why a 17-year-old is deemed to know significantly more than a 16-year-old, for example, but every society needs to choose where they draw the line on this. The law is there to protect younger people. This is one area where you need to know the law, because if you are 17 or older and you have penetrative sex with someone below the age of 17, you could face prosecution. And, like I said at the beginning of this chapter, you can be a victim of this crime too. Just to be clear on exactly what I mean by that, if a man penetrates you before you reach that age, he can be charged with what is commonly referred to as statutory rape. If a woman engages in sexual activity with you before you turn 17, she can be charged with sexual assault.

Let me explain it like this. Remember earlier in this chapter I really promoted the benefits of partners talking and listening? I said that as long as two people can openly express what they're comfortable doing and they respect what each other says, they're getting things right with regard to consent. This doesn't include people under 17, though, because according to Irish law they are not in a position to fully understand the consequences of their decisions or behaviour in this area. Therefore, verbal consent – saying yes to something – from someone under 17 is not going to protect you – or your partner – from being charged if you have sex. The law is the law!

It's really important to know the law, but it's also vitally important to know that every country has its own laws on this issue. Therefore, knowing that Ireland's age of consent is 17 is irrelevant if you're in Chile, for example, where the age of consent is 18. Remember, the only law that counts is the law of the country you're in, so make sure you know it!

IF IT'S NOT OK FOR ONE OF YOU, IT'S NOT OK.

Here are just a few examples of how differently this issue is handled around the world.

The age of consent is 18 in Nigeria, but it's 16 in the Philippines. It's 13 if you happen to be in Japan but it's 14 if you're in Germany, Portugal or Italy. Fifteen is the age of consent in Sweden, Greece and Croatia, whereas it's 16 if you're in the Netherlands or South Africa. Like in Ireland, the age is set at 17 in Cyprus. It's 18 in Turkey, 16 in South Korea, and it's 21 in Bahrain for unmarried people.

And, just to complicate things further, there's actually no age of consent for sex between unmarried people in Saudi Arabia, Yemen or Qatar. In those countries, all sexual behaviour outside of marriage is forbidden.

I hope you're beginning to realise the importance of knowing the law wherever you are. If you're unsure, just check the government website of the country you are in for the info you need. **The message here is really easy to understand and simple to follow – just find out the law of the land wherever you are and be sure to obey it.** And as long as you're in Ireland, you need to be aware that the legal age of consent to sex is 17.

HOW TO KNOW FOR SURE

Have you ever lied about your age to anyone? I know I certainly did loads of times when I was a teenager. If I wanted to rent an 'over 15s' movie from the video store (ask your parents!) when I was only 13 or 14, I always tried to blag that I was older than I was. If I wasn't convincing, I'd be going home without the film. Other times I tried to claim I was younger than I really was just to get away with lower bus fares. When I wanted to get cans at the weekend from the off-licence, but I wasn't old enough to get served, I'd often bring fake ID with me to trick the salesperson into thinking I was older. Other times I'd try to lie my way into pubs or nightclubs. In all cases, the main aim was to hide my real age from the people for my own gain.

Other than the video store example (honestly, they were huge back in the day!) examples like these might be pretty familiar to you or your mates. Your age has a pretty big bearing on what you can and can't do, which can often be hugely frustrating. I'm sure some days you're treated like a kid and other days you're expected to act like a grown-up. Some days you're given the freedom to act as you like and the next day, you're back to having to ask permission to go the toilet. It can be really annoying to be defined so much by your age, which is why so many young people exaggerate and lie about it.

When it comes to having sex or being sexually intimate with someone else, it's really important to know for sure that your partner is being honest. Obviously, it's equally important that you're honest yourself. During workshops, lads often say that there's no way of knowing that you're being lied to, especially because some people look older than they are. However, every time someone says this, other lads in the workshop immediately give suggestions on how to find out. These are the three most popular examples lads your age give to each other on how to make sure someone you've just met is telling the truth about their age:

- Check their social media pages for clues. Often pictures around birthdays or school events can help to reveal their true age, so scroll through them for clues.

- Keep asking questions. You may well know this from personal experience, but often people who are lying trip themselves up when you press them for further details of their story.

- If you know someone who knows them, or is in their social circle, you could discreetly check with them. This way helps to avoid any confrontation (remember, not everyone reacts well to the suggestion they're not telling the truth!).

Remember, this is one area where knowing the truth is vitally important.

CASUAL HOOK-UPS

Think back to the cinema example I used earlier in the chapter. That was my attempt to help you understand that working through differences in opinion and preference is a basic but really important part of any relationship. Sometimes it's to do with cinema trips, other times it's to do with choosing meals or where to go on a night out, but obviously you could apply it to any aspect of life where people can have different views. After a while together, however, couples don't need to keep having the same chats about the same topics because they will have a growing understanding of each other's opinions on loads of things.

The same applies to sexual activity and knowing each other's levels of comfort and pleasure. Very quickly, couples can learn about each other's turn-ons and turn-offs. In other words, when it comes to sex, people don't continuously ask the same questions of one another when they know for sure what the answers are going to be. Of course, this doesn't mean you automatically have someone's consent just because you know them well – not at all! – it just means that a couple can, over time, develop a deeper understanding of one another's preferences and comforts when it comes to sexual activity.

However, not all sexual activity is between people who are officially 'together'. To be honest, I don't even know what the proper definition of 'together' is anymore. I could spend pages and pages describing the different ways people relate to one another and describe the nature of their relationships, but I'll stick to a fairly basic description here – it's when two people see each other as their boyfriend or girlfriend and have an understanding that they won't be with anyone else. In situations like this, it's pretty easy to get to know what each other is comfortable with and interested in doing, but not every scenario is as straightforward as this.

Casual hook-ups happen all the time between people who don't know each other well. It might be at a party, in a club, at a pub or in someone's house, but these are the types of scenario where very little time is spent getting to know one another before things start to get sexual. At times like this, it's even more important to talk openly about how you feel about what you're doing because neither of you knows a bloody thing about the other. **In other words, the less you know someone, the greater the need to**

find out what each other is comfortable doing. And the best way of doing this, as you know by now, is to talk!

Check in with them to see whether they're OK and comfortable with what you are doing together. Keep in mind that they may not be enjoying things as much as you, and ask if that's the case. Hopefully they're going to be just as sound towards you and they'll be asking the same thing.

There are two big advantages to adopting this approach. Firstly, if your partner is not comfortable, it's better to know this there and then. It's too late to realise this the following day because it's too late to rectify anything. So, knowing for sure they're not comfortable gives you the opportunity of changing to something you both prefer. Secondly, and this is the part not many people realise, if you keep checking with your partner that they're enjoying what you're doing together, you've both got a much better chance of having an experience you'll both really enjoy. As I said at the start of this chapter, the more you talk with your partner, the better the experience is likely to be for you both!

DON'T BE A DICK

When it comes to sex and relationships, the more experience we get, the better we're all able to tell the difference between right and wrong behaviour. I cringe at some of the things I said when I was a teenager, but like most people, I learned from experience along the way. In other words, I got better at relationships the more practice I got.

For example, when I want to break up with someone, I don't ask my friend to tell my girlfriend for me. That was (possibly?!) OK when I was about twelve, but it's not great to behave that way when you're an adult. Also, I don't ask mates of mine to approach girls on my behalf in nightclubs to see if they like me. That was (borderline) acceptable in local discos when I was about thirteen or fourteen, but I wouldn't be happy if I was still doing that at the age I am now. In other words, there are certain behaviours which are OK when you're younger and which we all grow out of. This section, however, is not about those things.

The section is about the stuff that's never OK, regardless of your age. The stuff that everyone should know is bang out of order. The stuff that is wrong at every age and unacceptable in every situation. The stuff that is common sense to most people but, weirdly, still needs to be pointed out to some. This section is about helping anyone who needs help to *not* be a dick towards other people.

Before you read on, it's worth pointing out that this section is only relevant to a small minority of lads. Very few lads think it's OK to grope people in large crowds, or shout offensive things to people on the streets. Only a small minority of lads are complete dicks to other people, but this section is written especially for them. Because when it comes to discussing consent and learning how to do things right, it's often helpful to point out behaviour that is obviously wrong. You might quickly realise none of this behaviour applies to you, but you may well know someone who needs these things pointed out. If so, you'd be helping them out and keeping others safe by sharing some of the following points directly with them.

- If you grope someone or touch any part of their body without their consent, you're a dick!

- If you shout sexual things at anyone as they jog past in the park, for example, you're a dick!

- If your behaviour makes someone else feel sexually threatened or unsafe, you're a dick!

- If you ignore your partner when they say they want to stop during any kind of sexual activity, you're a dick!

- If you share sexually explicit footage of you and your partner without their consent, you're a dick!

- If you send nude images to someone without knowing in advance that they want to receive them, you're a dick!

- If you share any nude or partially nude images of another person without their consent, you're a dick!

- If you take advantage of someone who is really drunk and unable to properly consent to sexual behaviour, you're a dick!

- If you make a recording of you and your partner being intimate with one another without their consent, you're a dick!

- If you think any of the behaviour on this list is acceptable and that I'm wrong to call it out, you're a complete dick!

These aren't the only examples of behaviours which are completely unacceptable, obviously. In some of the ones I just listed, however, we could use different words instead of 'dick' to describe the person involved. In some cases, we could use the words 'sex offender'. In others, the word 'rapist' fits better. In many of them, words like scumbag, sex pest, sexual predator, deviant, pervert, and asshole would also work really well. If you are aware of anyone in your life who thinks it's OK to act in any of these ways, you would be doing them a huge favour by trying to ensure they never do.

WORKSHOP Q&AS

During consent workshops, the most interesting part for me is always the bit where lads give their opinions on how certain situations should be handled. I usually ask two specific questions to kick things off:

- **When two people are sexually involved with one another, which one gets to decide what exactly you do together?**

- **How do you know for sure your partner is consenting to what is happening between you both?**

Very rarely, if ever, does an entire room of teenagers give the same answer to either question. There is always a difference of opinion. Some people give the correct answer, and others give answers that are way off the mark. In all of the workshops, however, nobody is ever criticised for giving the 'wrong' answer. After all, the vast majority of lads in the workshop are sexually inexperienced and have had very few, if any, conversations with adults on this topic.

Teenagers can't be expected to know everything about this topic, but asking these questions gives everyone the opportunity to learn the right answer from someone else in the room. Here are some of the most common answers I get. Before you read my responses to each one, which answer would you give?

When two people are sexually involved with one another, which one gets to decide what exactly you do together?

THE OLDEST

I can see why some people would say this. After all, responsibility is often given to the eldest in certain situations. For example, isn't it normal for the eldest child to be put in charge of their younger siblings when parents have to leave? We're often led to believe that with age come experience and wisdom, or that we should 'respect our elders'. When it comes to consent and what happens between two people sexually, though, age isn't the deciding factor. Both people are completely equal when it comes to having a say in what they do together.

THE YOUNGEST

This answer usually comes from the assumption that older people will be up for anything, so it's therefore up to the younger person to decide how far things go. When it comes to sexual behaviour, though, you don't get to take charge because you're younger. You don't have greater say in what happens between you and your partner than they do. Whether older or younger, your age doesn't give you any more or less say on anything. Your body is yours, and your right to feel pleasure, comfort, safety and enjoyment is the same as everyone else's, but you don't get to have the final say on what anyone else does or doesn't do in the bedroom. It's entirely a two-way, mutual thing.

THE FEMALE

I hear this answer a lot! Many people assume that lads are always keen to go as far as possible, and that it's the girl's responsibility to either 'apply the brakes' or 'give the all-clear'. If you think that, it's understandable that you would assume the female gets to call the shots, sexually. However, and this can't be stated strongly enough, your biological sex does not give you any more or less say in what is happening between you and your partner. You have just as much right to comfort, safety and enjoyment as your partner, but neither you nor she has any right to take control!

THE MALE

If you're from one of those families where the father of the house is the authority figure, I could see why you'd say this. After all, you've been brought up witnessing a world where the man makes all the decisions, so this answer is understandable given your own life experience. It's really important not to get this wrong, however – when it comes to what two people do together sexually, nobody gets to call the shots or assume control just because of their biological sex. It doesn't matter what you hear from other people about the roles of men and women, or what you expect of yourself or other people based on their sex: when it comes to deciding what to do in the bedroom, both parties are 100 per cent equal and deserving of total respect.

THE PERSON WHO OWNS THE HOUSE

Some people think that what happens in their own home is their choice, or their responsibility. In some situations, that might be true. For example, you probably feel you're in charge of your bedroom – certainly more so than your siblings, anyway. You probably feel entitled to kick an annoying younger sibling out of your room if they're not doing what you want them to. This happens in lots of households, but it's important to realise that just because something is happening in a place where you usually feel in charge, this doesn't mean you're in charge of what happens sexually. Nobody is in charge! You and your partner have equal say in what occurs between you, and you should both feel entitled to be listened to and respected equally. In other words, it's completely a two-way street, wherever you are!

THE ONE WITH THE MOST SEXUAL EXPERIENCE

There are often scenarios in life where it makes sense for certain people to take charge. If you're lost (and have no access to WiFi), you'd ask someone who knows the area for directions. If your dog was sick, you'd take the vet's advice on what to do because they're the expert. There are loads of other scenarios where it's just common sense to let the person with most experience be the decision-maker. This does not apply to sexual activity, however. Regardless of how much experience people have in this area, nobody has the right to take charge of what another person does in the bedroom. Everyone has the right to make their own decisions based on what they're comfortable with, without having to justify or explain things to anyone else. Nobody is in charge in this area; everyone is equal.

YOUR BODY
IS YOURS,
NOBODY
ELSE'S. AND
NOBODY
ELSE'S BODY
IS YOURS.

NEITHER IS IN CHARGE – THEY'VE GOT JOINT RESPONSIBILITY

This is always true. When it comes to having sex, nobody has the right to consent on someone else's behalf, or make decisions for anyone but themselves. You don't get to do anything to or with anyone else's body without their full consent and agreement. Whether you know them a day or a decade, whether they're your friend or your spouse, whether you're drunk or sober – at no point do you get to make decisions without their say-so. **Your body is yours, nobody else's, and nobody else's body is yours.** If they're not consenting to sex, and you proceed to have sex with them anyway, it's no longer called sex. It's called rape.

How do you know for sure your partner is consenting to sex?

WHEN THEY INVITE YOU INTO THEIR HOME OR GO INTO YOUR HOME

I understand why some lads would say this. After all, I can think of countless movies and TV programmes where there's a scene at the doorstep when one person asks the other to come inside. There's usually this dramatic pause as if it's a really big question – like if they say yes, it's an agreement to something beyond simply going into the house. Often when they go inside, they get straight to it, too! It's important to separate what you see in films and what you expect to happen in real life. If your partner agrees to come into your house, or invites you into theirs, it shouldn't be taken as a sign they're up for sex. Maybe they just want to continue talking, have a few drinks, or use the bathroom! It's possible they do want to be sexual with you in some way, but there are lots of reasons why someone would ask you into their home, so never automatically assume someone is keen to have sex just because you go indoors together.

ONCE THEY GO TO A BEDROOM WITH YOU

So many people give this answer! Again, I think we can put this down to what we usually see in TV scenes. It's so common for scriptwriters of television shows to have sexual encounters happen in bedrooms. I assume you know this already, but sex can happen in plenty of places other than bedrooms! However, when people go into a bedroom together on television, it's often followed by scenes of a sexual nature. It's really important here to be sure you know that people go to bedrooms for lots of reasons – privacy, the desire to talk more, or maybe for certain sexual activity other than sex. Often – and this is kind of obvious when you think about it – they go because they want to sleep!

IF THEY REMOVE ALL THEIR CLOTHES

This is a really common answer, but I think we can blame television or porn movies for this one too. After all, being naked in porn usually means you're consenting to sex (in fact, every single type of behaviour in porn leads to sex!). It's not just in porn, though – being naked in regular movies is rarely just so people can talk or share meals together! What's really important to be aware of here is that making assumptions about someone's desire based on what they are or aren't wearing is going to create a lot of trouble for you both. It's entirely normal to feel comfortable enough with someone to be naked with them, without being interested or comfortable enough to have sex with them. In all cases, you've got to be sure what your partner is totally comfortable doing, and you certainly won't know for sure just by observing how much or how little they're wearing while they're in bed with you.

IF THEY'VE ALREADY HAD SEX WITH YOU BEFORE

This is a common answer. People can assume that, once you've had sex with your partner one time, you'll be having it all the time. In other words, every time you're intimate together, and the opportunity presents itself, you're going to be having sex. This isn't the case at all, though. Just because a person consented to a certain behaviour at a certain time – for example, having sex last Wednesday – it doesn't mean a thing when it comes to what they're comfortable or interested in doing with you in future. They may not have found it an enjoyable experience first time round, or perhaps they were in a specific frame of mind or mood that day. Actually, there could be loads of reasons why a person is up for doing something one day but not on another day, so you need to keep that in mind all the time. Consent is an ongoing thing – you've got to keep checking in with one another to make sure you're both entirely comfortable with what's happening in the present moment.

IF YOU KNOW THEY'VE HAD SEX WITH SOMEONE ELSE

I hear this a lot. Loads of people think that once they have a partner who is sexually active – particularly one who has already lost their virginity – this means their partner is automatically going to be keen to have sex with them as soon as the opportunity presents itself. Be very careful around this. There are loads of reasons why two people have sex with one another – length of time together, level of comfort and trust between them, strength of feeling for one another, influence of drink – so don't assume this means they automatically want to have sex with you too! Remember, the best way to avoid making assumptions that are way off the mark is to be open and communicative with your partner at all times. That's the only way to know for sure!

IF THEY SAID SOMETHING IN THE PAST ABOUT IT

This is one that trips up many people and in some ways it's easy to see why. Here's a common example – a couple agree to have sex the next time they're home alone together. Maybe one of them, say the girl in this example, said this after having a few drinks in a pub one night. Maybe she said it in a text, or whispered it in the cinema one night. Then, when the time comes, she feels differently. What seemed like a good idea last week doesn't feel so good today. And maybe she'd prefer not to go into detail about why she has changed her mind, but she just says she feels differently about it now. In those situations, it's so important to realise how she is feeling and be respectful of that. In other words, what someone said or agreed to in the past shouldn't be used to overrule their wishes in the present. Sex should only happen when there is consent from both people. People have a right to change their mind whenever they like when it comes to sexual activity.

FROM THEIR BODY LANGUAGE

Many people think they could read a person's body language and work out what they're thinking. The problem with this approach is that not everyone communicates in the same way using their body. Just because your previous partner moved their body in a certain way to communicate something specific, it doesn't mean your current partner means the same thing when they do the very same movement. It's difficult to gauge whether someone is consenting while in total silence, so it's always better to be as clear as possible. Give yourself the kind of advice we give to toddlers when we're unsure what they're trying to tell us – 'Use your words!' That way you'll find out how they're feeling about what is happening between you. And remember, there's far more to find out than simply whether your partner is OK with doing what you're doing. Letting each other know if you're enjoying it or not is also a really healthy habit to get into.

IF THEY DON'T OBJECT OR SAY NO

I understand why this answer is given a lot. Most people would work off the assumption that if their partner isn't up for something, they'd tell them. So, if they're not objecting, they must be silently OK with everything that's happening, right? It's easy to see why you'd think that. After all, how many times have you seen Hollywood movies depicting sex scenes between two people who remain silent throughout? It's like they're totally in sync with one another and have telepathic understanding of exactly what one another is thinking and feeling. When it comes to consent, though, it's vitally important to remember the following phrase – 'The absence of a no doesn't mean a yes!' Someone being silent isn't a sign of anything definite. This is because people can feel overwhelmed sometimes, and when they do, a common response is to freeze. When this happens, they're actually not able to say anything. It's really good advice to always look for a clear sign that your partner is comfortable and OK, and that they're enjoying what is happening between you when you're being sexually active with one another. So, a good rule of thumb is to always look for verbal consent – don't rely on your intuition or some of the other cues that are mentioned in this section. That's the only way to know for sure.

IF THEY SAY THEY CONSENT
This is how you know for sure your partner is consenting to have sex – or to engage in any other sexual activity for that matter – so the more you communicate openly with one another the better chance you'll both have of knowing how each other feels. And as I've said many times in this chapter, the more you know how each other is feeling, the better chance you both have of pleasing each other and enjoying the experience.

FREQUENTLY ASKED QUESTIONS

My questions about consent just kick things off. Pretty soon, the lads themselves are the ones looking for answers from me. Here are some of the ones I hear in virtually every workshop from lads your age.

OK then, you're saying to use words to know if someone is consenting. What words exactly?

There are loads of simple phrases you could use to let your partner know you're thinking about their levels of comfort and enjoyment when you're together. Things like 'Are you OK?' can be a bit waffly and vague. Asking, 'Are you sure you're comfortable/OK/ up for doing this?' gives very little room for mixed signals if it's answered properly – it's either a yes or a no! During consensual sexual activity it's then a good idea to check in with how both yourself and your partner are finding things. Doing this will help to improve the experience for you both. **The last thing you want here is the possibility of mixed signals or misunderstood signals and phrases, so be clear and open when speaking to one another.** It's worth remembering – if you're both constantly communicating to one another what you're enjoying and not enjoying, you're both massively increasing the chances of having a more enjoyable and fulfilling experience together.

In a nutshell, remember three things when you're with someone sexually.

- Check in with yourself on how it feels for you. *Am I OK with this?*

- Check in with your partner on how it feels for them. *Are you sure you're up for this?* If your partner consents, then proceed. If they don't, then STOP: don't ignore them, or try to convince them, or harass them ... just stop.

- If it doesn't feel OK for you, speak up. If you're being ignored, remove yourself from the situation as soon as possible because what is happening between you is sexual assault.

Aren't you going to really annoy your partner if every 30 seconds you keep asking if they're sure they're OK and comfortable and enjoying themselves?

I'm not saying you have to do it that often, but checking in with one another when a new behaviour is introduced would be a good idea (for example, oral sex, removal of items of clothing, a change in sexual positions). The thing is, the longer you and your partner are together the more you will be aware of each other's level of comfort in many different scenarios. The 'constant checking in' advice is useful in all scenarios, but especially in the early part of your relationship. Remember, the more a couple are aware of each other's level of comfort and enjoyment, the better the experience will be for them both. **In other words – the more communication, the better the sex!**

What's the story when alcohol is involved?

This is such an important question because this is when things can get very messy. Remember I said that once a person says yes clearly (or 'uses their words'!), you know for sure they're willingly consenting? Well, that was on the assumption that they're sober enough to know what they are saying and doing. When they're drunk, however, this whole topic becomes a little more complicated, and a lot less clear. The easy part is to refer to the law in this area – *a person incapacitated through drink or drugs is not in a position to give consent* – but applying that to real-life scenarios in a way that protects you and your partner isn't always straightforward.

I'll try to explain this in the simplest way possible. Let's take the most obvious example of someone who is way too drunk to respond properly to what's happening around them. Let's say they can barely stand up without someone supporting them. Let's be honest – living in Ireland you're going to witness this quite a lot! Having any kind of sexual interaction with them is completely out of order – you'd be clearly taking advantage of someone's total inability to protect themselves. Most people instinctively know the difference between right and wrong in these cases. So, in this case, even if the person clearly verbally consents (the main thing to look for in all other scenarios), common sense and decency tell you to ignore what they're saying and to acknowledge they're way too vulnerable for you to become involved with them.

The trickiest part is to realise that there are many grey areas here – namely, how drunk is too drunk to give consent? Everyone has a different threshold when it comes to alcohol tolerance, so it's no use quoting amounts or units of alcohol (for some people, one drink is too many!). The main thing here is to be super-aware that once your partner has consumed alcohol, you need to apply extra care to the whole area of consent and be extra considerate of their wellbeing. And that's going to be particularly tricky to do if you're drunk yourself! So, the main point to remember here is to be extra careful when there is drink in play. Ensuring you and your partner are safe and fully in control of what you say and how you behave will become a lot trickier if at least one of you is no longer sober.

It's the same with drugs. How often have you seen someone's personality, behaviour and mood completely change when they've taken drugs? They're really vulnerable to someone taking advantage of them, so the same rule of thumb applies here as it does when alcohol is involved – be extra considerate and thoughtful about whether it's right to be sexually involved with them in any way. Words of consent from someone who is really drunk or high should not be taken as a green light to get involved. In addition to the harm you'd potentially cause the person, you'd be putting yourself in a vulnerable position legally.

In a nutshell, if you have sex with someone who's too drunk or high to give their informed consent, you've committed rape.

Lessons from the therapy room

Sophia

Sophia was in her early twenties when she came to see me. Initially, she spoke about a family situation that was causing her some distress, but two or three months into our work together, she spoke about a traumatic experience she had endured over two years earlier. It had taken her every day of those two years to develop the capacity to speak about her ordeal, and she needed those three months in therapy to figure out if she was ready to say it to me. It was the most difficult conversation of all, about the most horrendous experience of her life. Sophia had been raped by someone she knew very well. Throughout our time working together, she spoke about how it impacted her feelings towards herself, her body, relationships and men. She described the impact it had on her behaviour, her sense of safety, her self-esteem and her mental health. She had twice attempted suicide. For the whole two years, she had been trying to outrun the trauma she had endured that night, without telling anyone what she was going through or what had been done to her.

Unlike some of the other stories from my therapy room, there is no need to appreciate nuance or circumstance with this one. Non-consensual sex is rape, and it can devastate people's well-being and their lives.

Lee

Lee came to see me on his own when he was 18. He began the first session by explaining the details of a very disturbing situation. He had been in a six-month relationship with Louise, who was two years younger than him. Louise's parents didn't approve because of their age difference. Her mum, in particular, constantly tried to convince Louise to break up with Lee. He and Louise were sexually active with one another from very early on in their relationship, but everything changed when Louise's mum walked in on them having sex in her bedroom. She kicked Lee out of the house immediately, and reported him straight away to the Gardaí for raping her daughter. Later that evening two Guards called to his house to bring him to the station for questioning. Since Louise was below the age of consent, Lee was being charged with statutory rape.

Lee came to therapy for almost eight months. The charges were dropped within a few months, but the whole episode caused huge upset to Lee, Louise and their families. When the risk of criminal proceedings had passed, we began to explore some of the issues raised by this case. Lee was aware of the age of consent, so too was Louise, but they were unaware of the consequences of ignoring it. I wondered what else he didn't know. It turns out his sex education was limited to what he knew from watching porn. He didn't have older siblings to advise him, nobody was educating him, and his parents thought sex was something people shouldn't discuss. I was struck by how avoidable it all could have been if Lee or Louise had been given appropriate guidance on this issue long before this happened. The big lesson for Lee was the importance of waiting until your partner has reached the age of consent. It doesn't matter how well you know them or how long you've been in a relationship with them. It doesn't matter how comfortable or enthusiastic they are to have sex with you, it's always against the law.

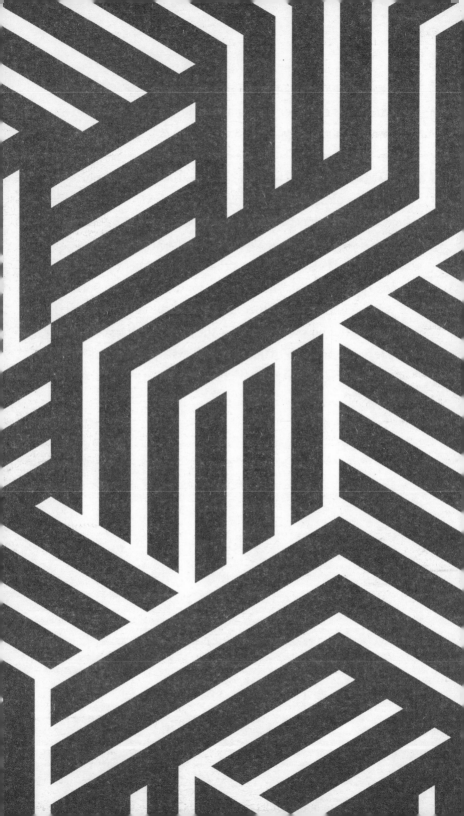

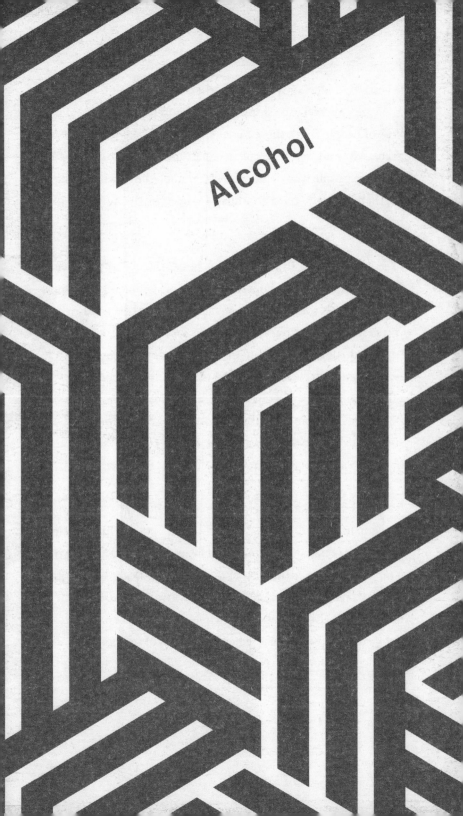

Alcohol

If you're wondering why there's a section on alcohol in a book about sex and relationships, you're almost certainly not alone. Lots of people think these topics should be kept completely separate. After all, many people in relationships don't drink, and there are people who drink who prefer not to be in relationships. So, there's a really good argument for keeping this topic out of a book like this.

I see it differently. In much of this book, the aim is to provide you with information about the realities of sex and relationships. The purpose is to help you make more informed decisions when you're in certain situations yourself. It's not about telling you what to do or criticising you for making poor choices, it's about helping you to have healthier and more fulfilling experiences as often as possible (spoiler: you are almost definitely going to make poor choices at some point!). And in order to do that properly, we shouldn't shy away from discussing the role that alcohol can play in this area of people's lives.

It's important to say that everyone has their own personal relationship to alcohol. You may already know what it's like to drink alcohol, or you may not. You might be looking forward to trying it or you may have no interest in the stuff at all. Regardless of how much or how little experience you have with alcohol so far, or how much or how little you go on to drink in your life, being aware of the factors that are in play when the worlds of relationships, sex and alcohol overlap is very important. That's why this chapter was included in a book like this.

I think it's really important that we adults are as open as possible with young people about the reality of alcohol and the impact it can have – both good and bad – on any situation. And, just to remind you, this is not going to be a lecture about the dangers of drink or an attempt to pressure you into being a non-drinker. Alcohol can be a positive addition to many situations for many people. You're going to make your own choices when the time comes, so it's not my aim to nudge you in any particular direction. This section is aimed at helping you to understand the ways in which alcohol can influence people and their behaviour. After that, it's entirely up to you what choices you make.

I won't be talking much about drugs here, but keep in mind that a lot of what I'll be saying about the impact of being drunk can also apply to situations where people have been taking recreational drugs.

Me and alcohol

Most young people in Ireland know at least one adult who drinks very heavily. It might be a relative, someone in the local community or a family friend. When I was a boy, my dad's drinking caused so much trouble for our family that it turned me off the thought of ever drinking myself. I took the pledge at my Confirmation, when I promised I wouldn't drink until I was 18, but really my intention was to never drink at all. Some of my friends started drinking as soon as we got to secondary school, but I wasn't interested. I had seen how damaging alcohol could be to a person so I didn't think I was missing out on anything. All I wanted to do back then was play football, so drinking really wasn't something that I felt I was missing out on.

Then, on a family holiday when I was 15, I decided to have a few cans myself. I had obviously stopped caring about the promise I made a few years earlier. A couple of years later, I left home to move to London on my own to be a professional footballer, and by then I was drinking every weekend. By the time I was 24, I was drinking so much so regularly that I would have very little memory of anything I said or did while I was drunk. I started to take drugs at that age, and pretty soon it would be fairly normal for me to take drugs with friends whenever we drank (which was very often!).

I realised my drinking was out of control when I was 32, so I gave it up altogether. **Some people can drink in a controlled, measured way, and it never causes them a problem, but I knew that wasn't me.**

I'm telling you all this because I don't want you to think this section is going to be a big long lecture about the dangers of drink and drugs. I am in no position to lecture anybody about this subject, so I don't. What I'm going to do instead is take you through all the ways in which alcohol and drugs can affect a person's thoughts and behaviour, and go through some of the specific ways it can impact relationships and sex.

Let's *not* talk about alcohol

Considering how prominent alcohol is in much of Irish society, you'd think we'd be really good at talking openly and honestly about all the ways it can impact people. You might think that, as a country, we have always been really good at supporting young people to learn how to have positive experiences with drink. You might assume we'd be really good at telling the difference between healthy and unhealthy drinking, for example, or that we Irish would be able to spot very quickly if we had a problem with drink ourselves. Unfortunately, things are a little more complex than that when it comes to drinking and discussing alcohol.

There are people who warn against the dangers of drinking, and then there are other people who refuse to acknowledge drinking can ever be a problem. Some people love it, others stay away from it, while some can take it or leave it. Even within your family you may notice your parents or other relatives think differently from one another on this topic. **You've probably already picked up a lot of mixed messages yourself about this, which can make it hard to know who to listen to or what to believe.**

I don't recall too many detailed chats about drinking when I was a teenager. It was something we weren't meant to do before reaching 18, so we were just warned off it. We didn't want adults knowing we were drinking, and adults wanted to assume we weren't, so it suited everyone to avoid the topic altogether. I remember hearing the odd 'Wait 'til you're old enough' speech from teachers in school, but I don't recall anyone sitting us all down and explaining the issues that can arise when people drink. Never once were there any discussions about how drinking can influence romantic or sexual scenarios. Back then, the only learning available to us was by making mistakes or getting into difficulties ourselves.

This chapter will help you to grasp some of the issues that arise when alcohol is involved, which saves you the hassle of having to make mistakes in order to learn.

A PERSONAL CHOICE

Whether you live in a home where drinking is very common or very rare, you are reaching the age when the choice to drink yourself will be all yours. The older you get, the more freedom you'll have to decide what to do with your own time. And, more importantly, you are at an age when the consequences of those decisions will be yours to manage.

The truth is that many teenagers make choices around alcohol that have nothing to do with what the law says or what their parents say (I have no doubt you know this already!). Most people make decisions based on what they feel is the best call for them personally. Often, and this is especially true with lads your age, people's decisions are influenced by their mates. In other words, teenage lads often turn to each other for guidance and direction on what to do, particularly when it comes to drink and drugs. So yes, it's a personal choice, but these aren't decisions people make alone.

IT'S REALLY IMPORTANT TO LEARN HOW ALCOHOL IMPACTS YOU.

Classroom discussions with teenagers about drink are always entertaining and insightful. Once everyone realises I'm not there to gather intelligence to report back to teachers or parents, we usually have some really honest and open chats about their decisions, opinions and behaviours around alcohol usually follow.

Here's some of the most common answers lads gave when we discussed the reasons for drinking on a night out:

- 'It relaxes me.'

- 'It's an escape.'

- 'To feel more confident.'

- 'To feel less anxious.'

- 'All my mates do it.'

- 'To feel less self-conscious.'

- 'To fit in.'

- 'To be able to chat to someone I fancy.'

Not everyone reacts the same to alcohol, but it's understandable why alcohol would be appealing to lads who give these answers. A lot of people, especially teenagers, feel self-conscious and unsure of themselves, so the extra layer of courage and confidence that comes with drinking can be very welcome. The tricky aspect of this, however, is that it's hard to control your reactions every time, especially at times when you drink more then you usually do.

If you drink on an empty stomach, for example, you may get a stronger reaction than normal.

While the amount you drink matters, if alcohol helps you to achieve the items on the list above without giving you any problems in other areas, you are likely to have a very healthy relationship with alcohol in your life. What is always noticeable in the workshops is how few people say they drink because they like the taste, which seems a little odd. Almost everyone who says they drink says they do it for the effect alcohol has on them, which makes it all the more important to be aware of the different ways it can impact people. **What I really mean here is that if you drink, or you think you'd like to drink, it's really important to learn how alcohol impacts you.**

Here's some of the most common responses to the question of why lads stayed sober on a night out:

- **'To stay in control.'**

- **'I prefer to be myself.'**

- **'Don't want to feel like crap the next day.'**

- **'Don't want to do something I'll regret.'**

- **'I've seen the carnage it creates and that puts me off.'**

- **'It's much cheaper!'**

- **'I'm very healthy/sporty.'**

These are all valid reasons why opting to remain sober is a perfectly understandable choice for someone to make on a night out. If these are your reasons, and staying sober works for you, there is no reason to be concerned about the impact of getting drunk or the pitfalls of drunkenness in this area.

However, even if you plan to always remain sober, this section is still important for you. As you know, most teenagers look to each other first for support, so being sober in a group that is drinking, you may be in the best position to help friends or partners of yours who run into difficulties in this area. Even if you never drink yourself, it's really worth educating yourself on all the possible issues that may arise in situations where alcohol is a factor.

ALCOHOL AND DATING

First of all, not everyone uses the word 'dating', do they? There are so many different words that people use when they talk about this topic (seeing each other, meeting each other, hooking up, etc.) that it would take too long to keep repeating them all throughout this chapter. I'm referring to those times where people are doing anything from flirting and getting to know each other to having sex – basically any scenario where people are *more* than friends with one another. So this section is about the different reasons that lads give for why they choose to drink or stay sober when they're on a 'date'.

You'll notice there's some similarities with the last section, but the big difference when it comes to dating is the presence of another person – your partner! **Given that alcohol can impact how we behave towards the people around us, it's important to be aware of the advantages of each option before you decide.**

Below are the most common reasons for why lads drink when they are on a date:

- 'It gives me confidence.'

- 'I'd feel too self-conscious if I was sober.'

- 'I develop the courage to make the first move.'

- 'I don't have any fear of rejection when I drink.'

- 'I don't doubt myself as much when I'm drinking.'

- 'I'm too shy without drink to talk to anyone so I need it.'

These reasons are all understandable. If you're someone who is quite shy, alcohol can seem to be a positive addition to a potentially romantic or sexual situation. It can also help to relax a person, while somehow also making them feel more courageous, two things which are very welcome if you're with someone you really like. This is often referred to as 'Dutch courage'. If these are your reasons, and you can achieve them without having any downsides, then it seems like your relationship with alcohol would be described as reasonably healthy.

And here are the most common reasons I've heard for why lads stay sober on a date:

- 'I can fully enjoy (and remember) the whole night.'

- 'I like to stay in control of what I say and do.'

- 'I don't want to embarrass myself.'

- 'I can look after my partner better if I'm sober.'

- 'I don't want to make a dick of myself in front of my date.'

- 'If I was messy like my mates, I'd get dumped.'

Like all the previous lists, these reasons seem perfectly valid. It would be hard to knock anyone for basing their behaviour on trying to achieve or avoid any of the things written here. It's also much cheaper to remain sober, and over time the money you'd save by not drinking regularly would go a long way to being able to afford to do things, go places or buy things you really want. One of the biggest factors to keep in mind on a date is the presence of your partner, so it's good that one of the reasons listed here is being considerate of them. **I'm sure the last thing you want to become is one of those lads who never considers how their partner thinks or feels, so it's a particularly healthy sign if you're already starting to consider the impact of your actions on those around you.**

SEX AND DRUNKENNESS

Before I explain how being drunk can impact people's behaviour in the bedroom, I want to point out something pretty obvious – drinking alcohol doesn't always lead to drunkenness. Loads of people limit their drinking to just one or two drinks at a time and they never lose control of themselves. They don't have to worry about losing their balance, slurring their words, falling over or wetting themselves. They don't feel the need to keep going until they're completely wasted, and they'll never be put in an ambulance and taken to hospital to get their stomach pumped. They won't spend any of the night slumped over the toilet getting sick and they won't wake up the following day with a pounding headache. Yes, loads of people can drink in a controlled way, but this section isn't about those people at all.

And I'll point out another pretty obvious thing here too – not everyone who is drunk ends up in bed with someone at the end of the night. Come to think of it, drunkenness can often be the specific thing that prevents this. **It's really common for drunkenness to cause disputes between partners or put an end to people's nights out together, but weirdly, it can also be the main reason people hook up with one another in the first place.** There are loads of different ways that being drunk can impact a person's night out, but this section is about how things will be affected in the bedroom. (Obviously, people have sex in loads of different places other than a bedroom, but I figured it's just easier if I stick to this particular location!)

The main point to keep in mind is that while you might have your own ideas on how you would or should act and behave in bed with a partner, there's very little chance of you being able to stick to that if you've drunk too much. This is because being drunk impacts how we make decisions. If you've ever observed someone drunk you've probably gathered that already, but what you might not know is exactly *why* this is the case.

The purpose of this book is to help you make calls about your relationship to sex by using a specific part of your brain – the frontal lobe. The frontal lobe is responsible for judgement and decision-making. We make sound decisions when our frontal lobe is activated. However, when we're drunk, we move to using the limbic part of the brain, which isn't great for decision making or problem solving. When we use our limbic brain, our response to most dilemmas is to shrug our shoulders and say that we don't care. **We become unconcerned about consequences, which is all well and good in the moment, but it can often leave us haunted with regret for our decisions when we sober up and come back to our senses.**

Let's look at how drink influences people in relation to sex.

Safer sex

When you are drunk, your hand–eye coordination will be all over the shop so it'll be harder for you to correctly use a condom. In fact, you'll probably be a lot less bothered about ensuring you have safer sex because your brain has lost some of its ability to care about the consequences of your actions. Your partner – male or female – might also care less about you using a condom before you penetrate them. In other words, you'll both be at much greater risk of an unplanned pregnancy or infecting one another with an STI.

Communication

You'll have less ability to take on board what your partner is saying (you'll understand this if you've ever tried to speak to someone who's hammered drunk!). You may have much less ability to speak in a way that your partner can understand (you'll definitely understand this if you've been in the company of someone who's a drunken, slurry-voiced mess!). Not being able to properly communicate with one another will obviously impact everything. You won't be able to tell if your partner is enjoying themselves, wants to change what you're doing or wants to stop altogether.

Memory

This is different for everyone, but it's very common for people to have a 'blackout' once they reach a particular level of drunkenness. This is where a portion of their night won't be stored in their memory for them to be able to remember the following day. They might get flashbacks now and again, reminding them of what they did, but most of that section of the night will be erased from their minds. Waking up without any memory of where you were for parts of the previous night can really freak some people out, but it's something that's entirely caused by the amount they drank.

Consent

In the same way that a 14-year-old, for example, does not have the capacity to consent to sex in the eyes of the law (because they're below 17), the same applies for a person who's hammered. If you penetrate someone (put your penis into their vagina, mouth or anus) who doesn't have the legal capacity to consent, you've just committed the crime of rape. It is crucially important that your partner has the capacity to consent to what is happening between you, but this is not always the case when they're drunk. If you're very drunk yourself, you may not be able to tell your partner's level of drunkenness or their ability to consent, so you are both in a really vulnerable position.

Decision making

A sober mind thinks very differently to a drunken mind. Your choice of partner, your decisions on how to behave, what you say, your actions in bed – these are all areas that are massively impacted if you're drunk. In addition to decisions around contraceptive use (as already mentioned), your feelings around whether or not to allow yourself to be filmed, for example, can change when drink is involved. Since a decision like this can have lasting consequences – intimate footage now exists! – you should always be aware of the impact and influence that alcohol can have.

Awareness

Imagine being so drunk you're not aware the bedroom door is open. Imagine being unaware people are watching you and your partner together. Imagine being unaware people are filming you or taking pictures. Being drunk impacts people in loads of different ways, but one of those ways is to significantly reduce their ability to know what's going on around them. You could be less aware of your partner's feelings or whether they're enjoying themselves (as I've already touched on earlier), but everything else could also be beyond your understanding. I'm sure you don't need me to point this out, but anyone who is so drunk they're unaware of what's happening around them is in a very vulnerable and unsafe situation.

Behaviour

You'd be amazed some of the things people say or do when they're drunk that they wouldn't dream of doing sober! Maybe you already have loads of examples of this from your own life. When it comes to sexual activity, however, behaving in ways that are out of character can be very disturbing and upsetting for some people. They may regret and be self-critical for what they did. Maybe they acted or spoke to partners in ways they never normally would, or they behaved in ways that caused them embarrassment or shame. It's a common experience for really drunk people to wake up the next morning knowing a list of apologies are in order, and it's solely as a result of the quantity they drank.

Erectile dysfunction

There can often come a point in a night where you've drunk so much that it's no longer possible to get an erection. Once this point arrives, there's nothing you can do. You can watch porn on your phone, drink water to sober up, try breathing exercises to relax – you can try every trick in the book, but unfortunately, you've gone past the point where getting an erection is going to be part of your night. Obviously, the lack of an erection is going to massively impact your options from then on. Loads of lads ignore this warning and have to learn for themselves the hard way. (Even though 'hard' is probably not the right word to use here!)

MYTHS ABOUT DRINKING

I've held many workshops with lads your age on this topic, and loads of my teenage clients talk to me about their questions, thoughts and experiences with drink. I think it's better to be really open about these things to help inform people of where they are going right or wrong. Some stories can be very funny and some questions can be really thought-provoking, but it's common for me to hear young people say things that are untrue, unhealthy or misguided about this topic. I particularly like hearing lads say things that are not true, because it gives me and the rest of the class the chance to put them right on certain issues or point out where they are wrong in some of their thinking. The workshops are always aimed at giving information that is helpful and useful so that lads can make more informed decisions in their own lives after they leave. Below are a couple of the biggest myths/misconceptions I've been told by lads your age. I'm including them in this section just to help you realise how wrong they are.

Myth no. 1 – If you're drunk, you can't really be blamed for anything you do. It's not your fault if you're hammered!

It's true to say you may not be fully in control of what you do when drunk, or that you could act in ways you never would while sober, but suggesting you are blameless for your actions is pretty ludicrous. If a drunk person punched me in the face, for example, do you think I'd just laugh it off? If they damaged my car, do you think I'd happily pay for the repairs myself? If they vandalised my property or sexually assaulted me, do you think the Gardaí would just shrug their shoulders and laugh it off as the harmless actions of someone who was entirely blameless? You'd better believe there are consequences to your actions when you're drunk, but – and this is the important part to understand – being drunk can often make you less aware of what those consequences may be.

As you now know, the frontal lobe of your brain has the job of keeping you tuned in to the future consequences of your current behaviour. That's the voice in your head that's like a supervisor, pointing out the likely outcome if you do certain things. It can predict how you are likely to feel in future based on your own behaviour.

For example, that voice tells you to mind your language when you're speaking to the school principal, or a match referee, or your grandmother. It'll advise you against confessing your love for the person you fancy in front of your whole class. It'll remind you that you there are parts of your personal life that you shouldn't post on social media for everyone to see, or that you shouldn't forward certain text messages to your parents. It's the reason you delete your search history too. It's always aware of your surroundings, and keeps you informed on how to behave appropriately. You mightn't always listen to it, obviously, but when you're really drunk, it'll become very hard to hear what it's saying. The limbic part of your brain will have taken over, which is why so many people do things that are completely nuts when they're drunk. **But even if you may be unaware in the moment what the consequences may be, you should realise that being drunk won't prevent others from realising what you've said or done.**

Please don't think bring drunk is an acceptable excuse for all behaviour, because it's not.

Myth no. 2 – If a girl is drunk, she shouldn't complain if something bad happens to her. She has to take some responsibility for her own actions.

It's true to say that we are responsible for our own behaviour, and if we get drunk, we are less likely to be able to protect ourselves from danger or tell the difference between risky and safe situations. Most people who understand alcohol can understand that. Often bad things happen to people when they are blind drunk. Because of poor balance, for example, they can fall and hurt themselves. Because of poor awareness, they can forget where they left their phone or their money. Because of poor judgement, they can put personal information on social media and regret it the following day. These are all examples of bad things that can happen people who are drunk, and that almost certainly wouldn't have happened if the person had been sober.

However, if 'bad things' refers to incidents like sexual assault or other sexual offences against the person, then it's a very different discussion. We're no longer talking about the understandable mishaps that can happen any one of us when we've drunk too much; we're talking about the illegal acts of someone else. We're talking about a person who is preying on the vulnerability of a girl's drunkenness and her inability to defend or protect herself. We're talking about a criminal act and the girl in this example is the victim. There is an enormous difference between having little sympathy for a drunk person who loses their balance and falls over, for example, and saying a drunken victim of sexual assault can't complain because they were drunk in the first place! Saying their drunkenness is the problem is suggesting you don't see the actions of the other person – the sex offender – as the problem. It's kind of like saying you see the girl's drunkenness as the real problem, and that sexual offences against drunk girls are a predictable result of girls drinking. This is a pretty messed up way of thinking!

When I question lads who say this in workshops, a really interesting conversation usually follows. In all cases, they're referring to sexual assaults by lads on girls, as opposed to scenarios where girls are the perpetrators or lads are the victims. Someone often suggests that most lads wouldn't be able to stop themselves if they encountered a helpless girl in a vulnerable position, which usually gets a strong, angry reaction from the rest of the class. Most lads who hear this view push back angrily against it, saying it's wrong to assume every male would act like a sex offender if the chance presented itself. The discussions can get very heated, but the outcome is the same every time: we reach agreement on one pretty straightforward idea: if someone sexually assaults someone else – whether the victim is drunk or sober – they are the one completely in the wrong.

TO BE REALLY CLEAR HERE:
If a person engages in sexual activity with someone who is not consenting, they are committing a crime. All of the blame and responsibility lies squarely at the feet of the perpetrator.

Please don't excuse the actions of sex offenders anywhere, regardless of how drunk or sober their victims were. And if you don't trust yourself to make good decisions around sex when you're drunk, maybe that's a wake-up call to look at your relationship to alcohol.

BE A MATE!

As you can probably tell by now, I'm not encouraging or discouraging you here when it comes to drinking. You're going to make your own choices, for your own reasons, and the consequences of those choices will be yours to manage. You're not a kid anymore, so I won't pretend you're still at the stage when you do as you're told by all the adults in your life. **There are situations, however, where you'll be in a position to help others manage the consequences of their choices. In other words, you'll be able to help someone who's too drunk to help themselves.**

This section is about helping you be a better mate when drink is involved. We've all been in situations where someone close to us could do with a word of advice. Sometimes they need some guidance on what to do or how to behave. Maybe they needed a gentle reminder on the difference between right and wrong. Perhaps they're in a situation where, as a result of the drink they've consumed, they're not in a position to help themselves. Perhaps, and this is the area I want to focus on now, they are in a spot of bother and they need a friend to intervene to keep them safe.

Sometimes it's possible to sense danger in a situation, even if you're not directly involved. In fact, there are plenty of cases where onlookers are in a better position to predict what's about to happen. I'll give you an example.

THE DIFFERENCE BETWEEN STEPPING IN AND STAYING SILENT CAN BE LIFE-CHANGING.

Imagine you see two three-year-old kids attempting to cross a busy road right next to you on the footpath. You could do nothing, of course, and just let them take their chances, but the likelihood is you'd feel compelled to hold them back. Imagine for a moment that you did nothing, and just stood and watched them walk onto the busy road on their own. If the worst happened, I assume you wouldn't be standing there shrugging your shoulders, thinking, 'Well, it was nothing to do with me, I didn't tell them to cross the road!' Saying, 'Wow, three-year old kids are so damn stupid sometimes!' is probably not going to go down too well with anyone either. I bet there would be some feelings of guilt or regret on your part, knowing that you could have done something to protect them from themselves but you chose to do nothing. I assume that even though you didn't tell them to cross the road and you weren't driving the car that hit them, you'd still be wishing you had acted when you could have so none of it would have happened.

Acting at the right time to help other people avoid trouble is what this section is about.

Like the example I just gave, there are times where it's really not acceptable to just watch a scene play out. Sometimes, particularly when alcohol is involved, there are situations that require an intervention of some kind. This is even more true when your mates are the ones involved. Acting responsibly towards them, especially when they're drunk, is one of the many ways you can help keep them safe from harm. I'm not saying you should take responsibility for what they do, I'm saying that thinking responsibly on their behalf is sometimes required. In other words, there are times when you really need to step up and be a mate!

If you're unsure what I mean, read through the scenarios below. All of these are real-life situations that young people I've worked with have faced. In some of them, a friend stepped in to help out, and everyone involved was really grateful that nobody came to any harm. In some, nobody said or did a thing to help out, which is a matter of huge regret for the people involved.

What do you think you would do if you were faced with each dilemma? **Would you step in to help your mate make the right decision or would you stand back and allow them to learn from their own mistakes?**

- You know your mate is over the legal limit to drive but she has offered to drive you and others home from a party. She thinks her driving ability improves the more she drinks.

- You see your slightly drunk friend go to a room with a really drunk girl at a house party. You saw the girl half-asleep on a couch earlier, too hammered to realise where she was.

- Your drunk mate is showing you nude pics of his ex and says he's about to forward them on to your other mates. He is still pissed off by the break-up and says he doesn't care if she finds out.

- You know your friend is planning to have unprotected sex with a girl he just met, and both of them are drunk. He just said he'll pull out so she definitely won't get pregnant.

- You see your mate mocking a group of older lads walking past. You know he's too drunk to realise the consequences of his actions. If they catch him, he's bang in trouble.

- Your 18-year-old mate is about to go to a bedroom at a house party with a girl you think is lying about her age. She says she's 17, but you're pretty sure she's only 15.

In each of these scenarios, just like the example I gave with the three-year-olds crossing a busy road, you are in a better position than the people involved to realise what could be about to happen. In each case, you'd have the perspective that your drunken friend wouldn't have. You can join the dots between what is about to happen and the possible consequences for your friend and the others. In every scenario, your drunken friend is just as vulnerable as the three-year-olds on the road, in that their ability to sense danger and protect themselves from harm has nearly disappeared. These are the kinds of scenarios where people need their friends to step in on their behalf and keep them safe. **In some situations, the difference between stepping in and staying silent can be life-changing.**

I won't say which of these scenarios worked out well and which didn't. In some of them, a friend intervened on time and nobody ran into any difficulty. In others, the people involved were left to face consequences that were catastrophic. The more I work with young people who talk openly about the situations they face, the more I realise how crucial it is that they have friends who watch their backs. This is especially true when drinking is involved. Regardless of whether you drink yourself or how you feel about your friends getting drunk, it's important not to miss opportunities to help them out whenever you can.

And just in case you're worried your friend will be unhappy with you for getting in their way, especially when it comes to things like going to bedrooms with girls or driving their own cars home, you've got to remember one thing – they're drunk! They might well be unhappy in that moment, but when they sober up, they will once again be able to understand the consequences of their actions and the potential danger of the situation. They'll be able to look back and see what could have happened if you hadn't stepped in, which should make them feel unbelievably grateful to you for keeping them safe. Remember, they're using the limbic part of their brains when they're drunk, but when they sleep it off, they'll be back using their frontal lobe and their perspective will be very different from there!

Lessons from the therapy room

Lucas

Lucas (22) was convicted of sexually assaulting a young woman on a night out when he was 19. He was too drunk to remember all the details of what happened but the CCTV in the venue captured the interaction on camera. It was reported in the local media so everyone in his area knew about it. He lost many friends as a result, and couldn't face going to college so he dropped out. He knew he wouldn't be welcomed back to his GAA club so he left. He had planned to go to the USA but couldn't because of his conviction. When he came to see me, he was really struggling. He figured he should limit his job search to ones that wouldn't bring him into contact with the public, but any opportunities ended as soon as his past came to light. He was anxious about getting into a relationship with anyone because he figured he would be dropped as soon as they realised who he was. He was stuck in a pit of self-criticism, shame, regret, embarrassment and pain, and feared he would spend the rest of his life feeling like this. He needed a lot of support to help him to adjust to and survive this new reality. It was too late to turn back the clock, obviously, but he knew his drunken actions had drastically changed the course of his life.

Joey

Joey was 17 when his parents brought him to see me. He had been drinking with friends in the local park a couple of months earlier. One of the lads in the group, who Joey barely knew, started shouting abuse at any female joggers in the area, using insulting sexual language. Joey had never done anything like this before, but before he knew it, he was joining in and doing the same. A man in a house nearby filmed it all on his phone and brought it to the Gardaí the following day. The Guards brought the footage to his school and the principal identified Joey as one of the culprits. His parents were furious, and Joey, more than anything, seemed really embarrassed.

He had no explanation for why he did it, and was genuinely full of regret. Even though he had gone drinking before, he said it was the first time he had ever done something like this. He was mortified even talking about it. He knew how wrong his behaviour was, and how upsetting or frightening it may have been for the joggers. More than anything, he seemed completely baffled as to why he did it in the first place.

What Joey hadn't realised was that, regardless of your personality, alcohol has the power to influence a person to act in ways they never would normally. He had no understanding at all that a person can do something completely out of character when they're drunk. What he also didn't fully appreciate is that lads of his age are often easily influenced by the behaviour of the people around them, particularly when they're in a group and they're drinking together.

So, not only does it matter *how much* you drink – but it matters *who you're drinking with* too. The Guards didn't pursue the matter, but he knew he had learned an important lesson the hard way: being drunk doesn't excuse anyone from the consequences of their actions.

John
While this chapter has all been about alcohol, I want to give you an insight into the role drugs can have.

John was 19 when his parents brought him to see me. He smoked weed daily, having tried it for the first time when he was 15. His parents constantly lectured him, accusing him of wasting his life. John said his parents were out of touch, and that they needed to educate themselves on how harmless weed really was.

'If anyone needs to change their attitude here,' said John to his parents, 'it's you two. You haven't a f*****g clue about life.'

I wondered how he was honestly feeling about things. For someone who said he had no problems, he seemed pretty miserable.

After a few sessions, when it was just myself and John on our own, he started to tell me that he didn't like the fact that all he was known for was being a stoner. He said nobody took him seriously anymore. He felt left out when his mates spoke about college and jobs because he had no plans for either. He couldn't go on holidays with them either because all his money went on weed. He left his GAA team a year earlier because he just lost interest, something he couldn't understand given how much he used to love it. But most of all, he said he felt lonely. His mates were all meeting girls and having relationships but nobody was interested in him, the guy who just smoked weed, mainly on his own, in his parents' back garden. He was becoming worried that he would be single forever, and would never have sex. He would often cry during sessions about how sad this made him.

Despite what he said to his parents about weed being harmless, he knew from his own experience that it wasn't true. He pretty much blamed his weed habit for everything that he was unhappy about in his life. He said it was like weed had caused a fog to descend over everything which stopped him caring about the people or the things that once mattered. Once he was able to admit this to himself, we were able to put our minds together to address his problem.

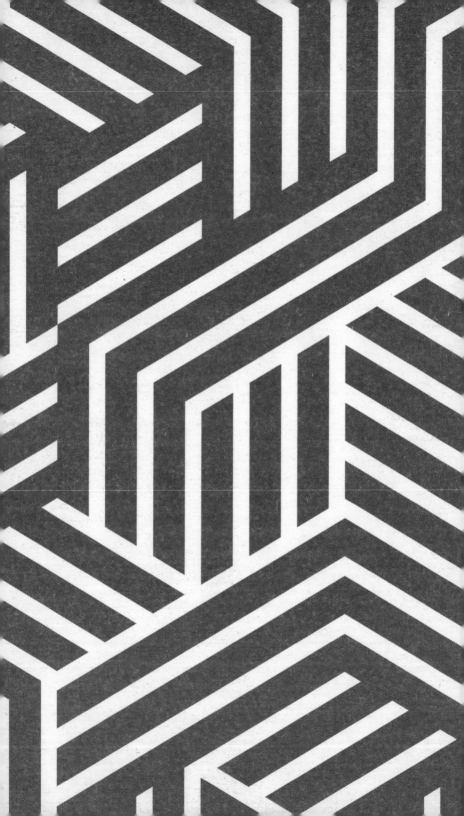

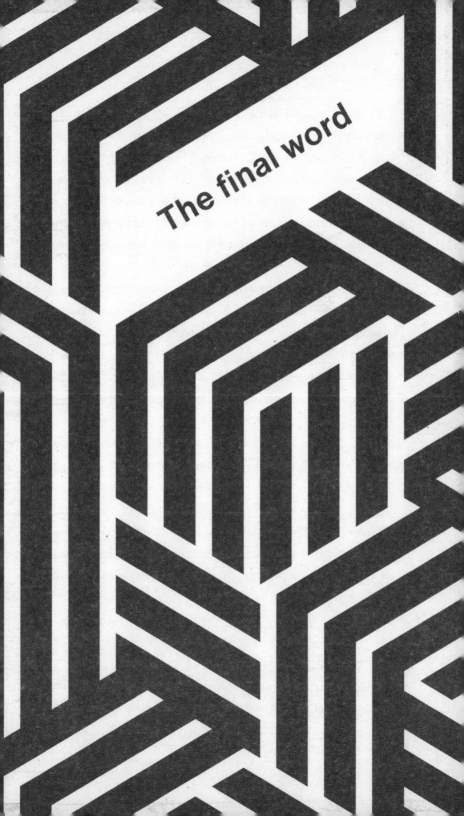

The final word

SUMMING UP

I hope this has been a useful guide in helping you to explore and understand parts of sex you might not have considered before. I hope it has helped you appreciate the richness and significance of your sexuality and how much fun, pleasure and joy it could bring to your life. **And if you're unsure about any aspect of sex or have a relationship concern of any kind, I hope you realise that discussing it is always a better option than staying quiet.**

We've covered many of the darker, uglier aspects of this topic also. If you weren't already aware, you now know how much trouble can be created by poor decision-making. It's just as important to understand the potential pitfalls of impulsive or thoughtless sexual behaviour as it is to know the rewards of doing things right. You should now be in a much better position to be able to grasp both.

Just like I did, you'll look back in future years on this period of your life and reflect on your decisions and actions. Like every adult I know, there will be some things you wish you had done differently. It's impossible for you to gauge how your older self will view these years and the experiences you have, but in the meantime, the best approach is to thoughtfully consider the impact of your behaviour rather than simply indulging every sexual impulse that comes your way.

YOUR MENTAL WELLBEING

Like everyone in their mid-teens, you're experiencing rapid and radical personal growth and change. While one of your 'jobs' as an adolescent is to work out who you are and how you'd like to express yourself sexually with the world, it's clearly not the only area of your development you need to look after. Your own mental health also needs your attention.

You may already tend to your physical health by exercising. Presumably you tend to your dental health by regularly brushing your teeth. I've covered the topic of your sexual health and how to look after it in the 'Safer Sex' chapter, but did you know your sexual behaviour and decision-making can impact your mental wellbeing?

It's not often spoken about, but our sexual choices and actions can have a significant impact on how we feel about ourselves and our lives. It's pretty obvious when you think about it, but behaving in ways that cause you trouble or distress is going to impact your mental wellbeing. It might be helpful at this point to bring you back to some of the examples I've already shared from my therapy room.

Think back to Freddie (page 44), who was infatuated with sex and didn't care how his behaviour impacted his partners. How do you think it made him feel about himself to constantly receive messages calling him a 'piece of s**t' (and far worse!) from ex-partners? He felt regret and guilt all the time, and it impacted his self-esteem and his confidence. A couple of his closest friends also dropped him because of his behaviour, which made him feel even worse.

Imagine what it's like to be in Adam's head (page 27). He had chosen to keep a fundamental part of himself hidden from the world and was stuck in a relationship with a woman despite being gay. He was angry at himself and the world around him all the time, and lived in fear of anyone finding out about his affairs with other lads. He felt trapped and alone all the time.

Imagine being in Toby's shoes (page 96). He was trying to somehow focus on his Leaving Cert, while coming to terms with an unplanned pregnancy and all the pressure and responsibility of becoming a teenage dad. He constantly berated himself for being in this position and was feeling completely overwhelmed all the time. It wasn't great to be Stephen either (page 97). He was trying to keep his STI private from everyone but he was too embarrassed to get it treated. He felt isolated and alone because he couldn't get with any girls, and he was terrified his friends and everyone in the area would find out what was wrong. Both Toby and Stephen ignored advice around protection and contraception and were struggling to deal with the direct consequences of their decisions.

Alan's mental health suffered a great deal too (page 61). He knew someone had explicit images of him and fully expected to get a call about it any day. You can imagine how this completely took over his mood. His was in a constant state of fear, panic, embarrassment, regret and shame. When I first met him, he said found it almost impossible to relax or focus on anything else.

And remember Lee, who was sexually active with his 16-year-old girlfriend (page 164)? He was so distressed by being charged with statutory rape and the prospect of being convicted that he attempted suicide. Thankfully he survived and arrived for therapy the following week, but the experience had a serious and long-lasting impact on his mental wellbeing. This was the result of ignoring the laws around the age of consent. The time I spent working with him is one of the main reasons I decided to write this book and support young people in this area.

All of these examples should help to illustrate a very important point. Our experiences in this area – particularly the negative ones – can have a significant impact on our mental health. They can be the cause of so much mental anguish and distress. That's why it's so important to box clever. It's so beneficial to think smart. **You might not have heard it phrased like this before, but being clued in when it comes to your sexual behaviour and decision-making can help protect you from experiencing additional challenges and difficulties with your mental wellbeing.**

In other words, there's a strong link between good sexual behaviour and positive mental health. Your sex life has the potential to make you feel great about yourself and seriously improve your self-esteem. While I'm sure you hope to avoid ever feeling similar to the lads I've just mentioned, if you find yourself in need of support or just someone to talk to, it's important to know you have options.

TIME TO TALK?

There are many different reasons you may choose to speak to others about your personal life. You might be facing a difficult dilemma, for example. Maybe you have to make a decision and you're not sure whether to trust your own judgement. You might be reeling from an experience that didn't go well and you've realised it has really impacted your mood. You could have doubts about how you should handle an ongoing situation or you might want someone's reassurance that things will work out. It's really healthy to want to talk to someone or to seek support for what you're going through, but it's just as important to choose well when you're deciding who to approach.

At the very beginning of this book, I said that I wanted you to realise the value of talking while being mindful of guarding your own privacy. **In other words, while it's good to talk, it's also important to talk to the right person at the right time.**

Some of the sexual experiences we have are not ones we would like our entire social circles to learn about, so it's wise to choose carefully. You mightn't be comfortable opening up to a parent either, for obvious reasons. In some cases, the privacy of someone else (for example, your partner) would be impacted if you spoke openly about certain situations. This is where speaking to a complete outsider such as your GP or a therapist would be really useful. You wouldn't have to worry about anyone else finding out because these professionals are required to keep what you say confidential, and you're in the hands of people who are specifically trained to know how to support you.

If you get to a point where you would like to speak to a therapist, below is a list of some organisations that can help. **If you want to speak about a sexual experience that has caused you distress or difficulty, there are organisations that provide the kind of specific support you may be looking for.** Even if none of these seem relevant to you now, it's good to be aware of these options in case someone you know comes to you looking for help.

GETTING SUPPORT

Counselling & psychotherapy

BLACKFORTINSTITUTE.IE
Not all psychotherapists have received training to work with young people, but Blackfort Institute's website contains a list of psychotherapists working all over Ireland with expertise in working with adolescents.

CARI.IE (OR CALL 0818 924567)
CARI provides therapy for children and adolescents who have been affected by sexual abuse.

IAHIP.ORG
IAHIP's website contains a database of psychotherapists working throughout Ireland.

IACP.IE
IACP's website contains a list of counsellors and psychotherapists working throughout Ireland.

ONEINFOUR.IE
Professional counselling services for adults who have survived childhood sexual abuse.

RAPECRISISHELP.IE

This website provides information about the professional support and choices available to survivors of sexual violence. You can call the 24-hour helpline on 1800 778888.

Resources & supports

SEXUALWELLBEING.IE

This website provides relationship and sexual health information for Irish teenagers, and gives details of free home STI tests available to people aged 17 and over.

JIGSAW.IE

Jigsaw provides free, confidential mental health supports for young people aged 12–25. Check out their website for more details.

FOROIGE.IE

Foróige is a youth organisation that provides services and support for young people aged 10–18 all over Ireland.

SPUNOUT.IE

SpunOut is a youth organisation that helps young people understand the importance of wellbeing and how to maintain good health – physically, mentally and sexually.

Services

GUIDECLINIC.IE/STI-CLINIC/YOUNG-PERSONS-CLINIC

For people under 20 years of age, this a free service in St James's Hospital, Dublin, that provides STI testing, treatment and sexual health information.

MYSEXUALHEALTH.IE/YOUTH-HEALTH-SERVICES

For people under 23, the Youth Health Service is a free, non-judgemental sexual health and counselling service in Cork.

AISEIRI.IE

The Aislinn Centre in Kilkenny is for adolescents who require residential treatment for addiction.

PIETA.IE

Pieta House provides free one-to-one therapy to people in suicide distress, those who engage in self-harm, and those bereaved by suicide. Freephone 1800 247247 or text HELP to 51444.

SAMARITANS.ORG

If you feel like you need someone to talk to, you can call Samaritans for free, any time day or night, on 116123.

TEENLINE.IE

Teenline is an active listening service for anyone under 18. The number 1800 833634 is operated 24 hours a day, all year round.

CHILDLINE.IE

Childline can be contacted by any child or young person by calling 1800 666666, texting to 50101 or chatting online at Childline.ie 24 hours a day, every day.

MENSAID.IE

Men's Aid Ireland is a charity dedicated to supporting men and families subjected to domestic abuse. Call their confidential helpline 01 5543811 or email hello@mensaid.ie.

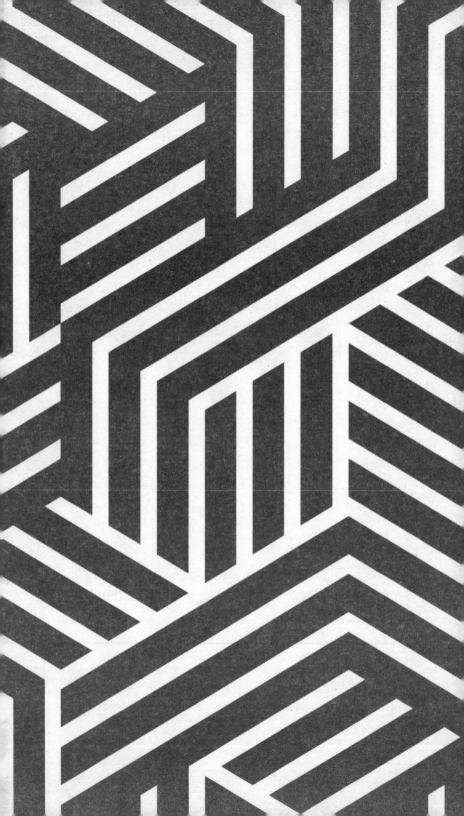

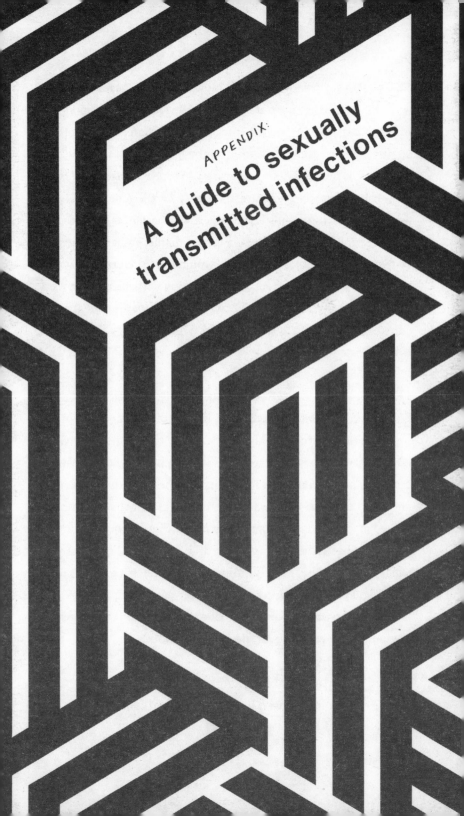

APPENDIX:

A guide to sexually transmitted infections

This section is a description of the most common STIs for those of you who want to learn more about this. You've been given enough information on how to reduce the risks in the 'Safer Sex' chapter, so this is just a rundown of some of the facts about each type of infection. It probably won't surprise you to learn that conversations about STIs were very rare in the past. People generally shied away from talking openly about personal experiences of successfully treating symptoms due to a mix of shame, embarrassment, or fear of judgement. Most people would have preferred to stay silent rather than share helpful information with each other. As you know by now, I'd much rather we informed one another about supports and treatment that can help, which is why I've included this information here.

The truth is that, while STIs are unwelcome, they are common. Effective treatments are available. No matter what your symptoms are or how you feel about discussing them with your GP, remember that they will have seen it all before. If you have any concerns about your own health in this area, get the problem checked out as soon as possible. It's better to get something looked at and treated immediately rather than sitting at home worrying that something is wrong and doing nothing about it. You'll be able to find details online about home STI testing kits which you can get delivered (in discreet packaging!). **Getting tested and treated has never been easier, so if you have any concerns whatsoever, don't hang about!**

I'll start by stating the blindingly obvious first – you can't get an STI from someone who doesn't have one. If your partner is sexually healthy, you don't have anything to worry about. An STI can be only be passed from an infected person to another person through skin-to-skin contact or through sexual contact.

There are three different forms of infection. You could have a *viral infection* (such as genital herpes, genital warts, hepatitis B, Human Immunodeficiency Virus (HIV)), a *bacterial infection* (for example, chlamydia, gonorrhoea, syphilis) or a *parasitic infestation* (such as pubic lice, scabies, or trichomoniasis).

FREQUENTLY ASKED QUESTIONS

Before I outline the details of each infection below, here are some of the most frequently asked questions teenagers have about STIs.

How do I know for sure my partner is sexually healthy?

There's no way of knowing for sure if your partner is clear of infection just by looking at them, because some STIs (like chlamydia, for example) can have no symptoms. Therefore, your partner – and even you! – could be infected and not realise it. The only way of knowing for sure either way is by getting a test at an STI clinic or from your local GP.

How do I make sure I don't get infected?

Using condoms is the best way to reduce the likelihood of getting infected, but unfortunately, they won't protect you entirely. You could still get certain infections (genital warts or herpes, for example) through skin-to-skin contact. The only way to guarantee not getting infected is to abstain from sexual activity and skin-to-skin contact entirely.

If I do get an STI, what happens then?

It depends on what infection we're talking about, but all infections are treatable with medication. Some are curable, and some, like HIV, are not curable but are treatable. Your GP or the doctors at the STI clinic will be able to prescribe medication, so the best thing to do is to book an appointment to see them as soon as you can.

Can I get an STI the first time I have sex?

Yes, absolutely. If your partner has an infection, they may pass the infection on to you, whether it's your first time or not. And remember, your chances of being infected greatly increase if you have unprotected sex.

What kind of STIs am I most likely to get?

According to the HSE, the three most commonly reported sexually transmitted infections in the 15–24-year-old age group are chlamydia, gonorrhoea and genital herpes.

THE MOST COMMON STIS

Here are the symptoms (for males *and* females) and the treatments of some of the most common STIs, with reminders of the specific ways you can protect yourself against acquiring them. You can still get infected even if you take precautions, but this section will be of particular use to you if you prefer to ignore the risks and take your chances instead.

Chlamydia

This is a bacterial infection. It is one of the most common and curable STIs.

IT MAY BE SPREAD BY:

- Unprotected oral, vaginal or anal sex (ejaculation does not need to occur)

- Close or intimate genital contact

- Unprotected rimming (mouth to anus contact, oral–anal sex)

- Touching an eye with infected fingers

- Transmission from mother to baby during childbirth

SYMPTOMS:

A person can have chlamydia and not have any symptoms. It is often referred to as 'the silent infection', as most infected women, and about half of infected men, will not experience any symptoms. As symptoms may not be present, the only way to know if a person has a chlamydia infection is to have an STI test.

If a person does have symptoms, they usually start to develop between one and three weeks after infection. They may include:

- Inflammation of the rectum/anus, vagina or urethra

- Burning/discomfort when urinating

- Abnormal discharge

- Bleeding between periods

- Bleeding or discomfort after sex

- Discharge from penis

TREATMENT:
Chlamydia is treated with antibiotics.

PROTECTION:
You can protect yourself by using a condom correctly every time you have sex – including oral sex.

Gonorrhoea
This is a bacterial infection.

IT MAY BE SPREAD BY:
- Unprotected oral, vaginal or anal sex (ejaculation does not need to occur)

- Close or intimate genital contact

- Unprotected rimming (mouth to anus contact, oral–anal sex)

- Touching an eye with infected fingers

- Transmission from mother to baby during childbirth

SYMPTOMS:
A person can have gonorrhoea and not have any symptoms, so you'd need to take an STI test to be sure you don't have this infection. For those who show symptoms, they usually develop between one and fourteen days after infection, and may include:

- Sore/inflamed throat

- Burning/discomfort when urinating

- Abnormal discharge from the penis/vagina/anus

- Bleeding between periods

- Discomfort during or after sex

TREATMENT:

Gonorrhoea is treated with antibiotics. It is important to note that, left untreated, gonorrhoea can cause serious and permanent health problems in both men and women, including infertility.

PROTECTION:

You can protect yourself by always using a condom every time you have sex – including oral sex.

Genital herpes

This is a viral infection. It is caused by the herpes simplex virus (HSV). There are two types:

HSV-1 usually affects the mouth and causes cold sores. However, it can be spread to the genitals through oral sex.

HSV-2 usually affects the genitals.

IT MAY BE SPREAD BY:
- Direct skin-to-skin contact

- Unprotected oral, vaginal or anal sex (ejaculation does not need to occur)

- Unprotected rimming (mouth to anus contact, oral–anal sex)

- Transmission from mother to baby during childbirth

SYMPTOMS:

A person can have herpes and not have any symptoms (which underlines the importance of having protected sex at all times).

When they do occur, symptoms usually appear between two and twelve days after infection and may include:

- Flu-like symptoms, such as discomfort or fever

- Blisters or ulcers that can be itchy and appear externally on genitals and/or rectum. After these blisters break, they may be painful, but will heal over in seven to ten days.

- A burning sensation when passing urine

TREATMENT:

Herpes is treated with prescribed medicine to reduce discomfort during an outbreak. The virus stays in your system and may cause further outbreaks. Subsequent outbreaks are usually less severe.

PROTECTION:

Avoid intimate contact with anyone who is infected. And given the difficulty in knowing for sure if someone is infected, ensure you use a condom every time you have sex, including oral sex.

Genital warts

This is a viral infection. It is caused by certain strains of the human papillomavirus (HPV). It is a very common STI.

IT MAY BE CAUSED BY:

- Unprotected anal and vaginal sex (and sometimes oral sex, although this is rare)

- Intimate/close genital and skin-to-skin contact

- During childbirth, HPV can be transmitted from mother to child if the mother's infection is active.

SYMPTOMS:

A person can have the human papillomavirus and not have any symptoms. Some people will not be aware that they have HPV. It can be passed unknowingly from one partner to another, and it can take up to a year for warts to appear.

The most common symptoms, when they occur, are:

- Painless fleshy lumps around the vagina, penis, anus, scrotum, tops of the legs (basically, anywhere on the genital area)

- The warts can be raised or flat, single or multiple, or appear in clusters. They can be small or large.

- Warts can settle by themselves without treatment, but the virus will still be present, and it can still be passed on.

- Symptoms can recur, and this varies from person to person.

TREATMENT:

There is no cure for the virus that causes genital warts. However, most people with a healthy immune system can clear or suppress the virus over time. The aim of treatment is to remove any visible warts, and this can be done in a number of ways, depending on their location, size and the number of warts present. Following diagnosis after a visual examination of the genital area by a nurse or doctor, the following treatments are available.

- **Lotion/ointment by prescription**

- **Removal by freezing/burning**

- **Laser treatment**

The HPV vaccine protects against genital warts, cervical cancers and other cancers.

It is important to note that a person can carry the virus, pass it on to a sexual partner and not have any warts themselves.

PROTECTION:

Although it's not 100 per cent effective, using a condom offers the best protection against genital warts.

Pubic lice

Also called crabs, these are similar to head lice: tiny insects that live in body or pubic hair.

THEY MAY BE SPREAD BY:

- Close body contact with an infected person

- Infected bed linen, but this is very rare

SYMPTOMS:

- Itchiness in your pubic area that continues and worsens

- The lice may also be visible.

TREATMENT:

- Creams and lotions are available from pharmacies to treat infestations of pubic lice.

- If infected, it would also be advisable to have an STI check.

PROTECTION:

- Do not have intimate sexual contact with an infected person because condoms are unlikely to protect you from pubic lice.

Scabies

Although not considered a sexually transmitted infection, scabies can be passed on through sexual contact.

IT MAY BE SPREAD BY:

Scabies is caused by parasitic mites that burrow under the skin and lay eggs. It is usually passed on from one person to another by skin-to-skin or sexual contact. Scabies can live outside the body for up to 72 hours, and be passed on from clothing, towels or bed linen, although this is rare.

SYMPTOMS:

- It can take up to six weeks to notice symptoms after coming into contact with scabies. An intense itch, especially at night or after taking a warm shower, is noticeable.

- Also, silvery lines appear on the skin and between the fingers.

- A red itchy rash may also be visible. But this can look similar to other rashes and itchy skin conditions such as eczema, making it difficult to diagnose.

TREATMENT:

Scabies can be treated with a shampoo, cream or lotion that is left on overnight. Your sexual partner(s) and those in your household should also be treated, even if they don't have symptoms.

PROTECTION:

Do not have skin-to-skin or sexual contact with an infected person.

Trichomoniasis

Also known as 'trich', this is a sexually transmitted infection caused by a protozoan, a tiny parasite that is like bacteria. Most cases are found in women, although it can also affect men.

IT MAY BE SPREAD BY:

- Intimate genital contact

- Unprotected oral, vaginal or anal sex

- Transmission from mother to baby during childbirth

SYMPTOMS:

For women symptoms may include:

- **Vaginal discomfort**

- **An offensive smell**

- **Abnormal discharge**

- **Stinging or a burning sensation when passing urine**

For men these may include:

- **A rash on the penis**

- **Discharge from the penis**

- **Stinging or burning sensation when passing urine (although this is rare)**

- **Soreness around the foreskin**

While some people may not have any symptoms, they can still pass the infection on to a sexual partner.

TREATMENT:

Trichomoniasis is treated with antibiotics.

PROTECTION:

Using condoms correctly every time you have sex will reduce your risk.

HIV

The human immunodeficiency virus, known as HIV, attacks the immune system, weakening its ability to fight disease and infection. If not treated the virus may progress to Aids (Acquired Immunodeficiency Syndrome). Aids causes the immune system to break down, making the body unable to fight off certain infections.

IT MAY BE SPREAD BY:

- **Unprotected vaginal or anal sex with someone who is HIV-positive and not on effective HIV treatment**

- **Unprotected oral sex with someone who is HIV-positive and not on effective HIV treatment, although the risk is very low**

- **Sharing needles or other drug-using equipment with someone who is HIV-positive and not on effective HIV treatment**

- **Transmission from a mother to her baby during pregnancy, birth or breastfeeding if the mother is HIV-positive and not on effective HIV treatment**

- **Receiving contaminated blood products (although this is unlikely in Ireland, as donated blood is tested for HIV)**

SYMPTOMS:

Many people are unaware they are infected with the virus, as they may not feel sick for a number of years afterwards. That is why it is important to be tested if you have been at risk of contracting the virus.

Some people have flu-like symptoms when they are first infected. Over time, the virus's attacks on the immune system may lead to repeated infections and other illnesses. But the only way to find out if HIV is the cause is to have a HIV test. This is especially important for those who are at higher risk, such as men who have sex with men, or people who inject drugs.

TREATMENT:

HIV can be managed effectively with prescribed medications that work by preventing HIV from reproducing in the body. When taken properly, medication eliminates the chance of a person living with HIV passing the virus on to someone else. As there is currently no cure for HIV, treatment is lifelong, and enables most people with HIV to live long and healthy lives.

If you think you may have been recently exposed to infection, visit your GP or nearest STI clinic as soon as possible. Treatment for people who may have been exposed to infection is available, called PEP (post-exposure prophylaxis). This must be started within 72 hours of exposure to HIV and the treatment lasts for 28 days.

PROTECTION:

Always use a condom correctly before the penis comes in contact with the genitals or anus. Do not share needles or other drug-using equipment with anyone else.

Treatment to prevent infection, called PrEP, is available to protect people prior to exposure to HIV (including before sex). This is available through the HSE, but only to people who are HIV-negative.

Syphilis

Syphilis is a bacterial infection.

IT MAY BE SPREAD BY:

- Kissing an infected person

- Skin-to-skin contact that causes direct contact with a syphilis sore

- Intimate genital contact

- Unprotected oral, vaginal or anal sex

- Transmission from an infected mother to her baby during pregnancy

- Infected blood during a transfusion (this is very unlikely in Ireland due to donor testing)

SYMPTOMS:

Some people have no symptoms. It is important to be tested if at high risk (especially men who have sex with men). There are three stages to the infection.

- **STAGE 1:** Primary infection. This stage lasts between 9 and 90 days, which is the time it can take from first exposure to the appearance of the first symptoms. However, symptoms usually appear three weeks after infection and may include an ulcer in the mouth, genital or anal area.

- **STAGE 2:** Secondary infection. This stage lasts between six weeks and six months. At this stage, symptoms may include a red, spotty rash that usually appears on the palms of hands and soles of feet, but can appear elsewhere on the body.

- **STAGE 3:** Tertiary syphilis. This stage can occur months or even years after initial infection. It is very rare for the infection to advance to this stage. However, if it does, symptoms will depend on what part of the body it has spread to. These can include the skin, eyes, bones, blood vessels, heart and brain.

TREATMENT:

If syphilis is not treated, there is the possibility that it will lead to long-term damage to the eyes, heart, brain and nervous system. Tertiary syphilis may be fatal. Syphilis is diagnosed by a blood test, usually in an STI clinic, and can be treated and cured with antibiotics. Treatment will depend on symptoms and how long the infection has been in the body.

PROTECTION:

Condoms, when used correctly, can provide good protection from infection.

Hepatitis B

This is a viral infection that affects the blood and liver.

IT MAY BE SPREAD BY:

- Unprotected oral, vaginal or anal sex

- Unprotected rimming (contact between the mouth and anus)

- Sharing drug-using equipment with an infected person

- Transmission through blood and other body fluids

- Transmission from an infected mother to a baby during pregnancy or childbirth

SYMPTOMS
- **Tiredness**

- **Nausea/vomiting/diarrhoea**

- **Flu-like symptoms**

- **Fever**

- **Jaundice (yellow tinge to eyes and skin)**

- **Itchy skin**

TREATMENT
Following diagnosis by blood test, treatment is available. There are different stages of hepatitis B infection, some of which need treatment. Other stages require regular monitoring rather than treatment.

PROTECTION
- **There are vaccines to prevent the infection.**

- **Don't share needles.**

- **Always use a new condom correctly and put it on before having sex.**

Acknowledgements

This book is the culmination of years of work I could not have done without the expertise, guidance and support of many others. In no particular order, I'd like to thank them here.

To the staff at St Benildus College, Kilmacud, particularly former principal Martin Johnson and former deputy principal Oisín McKeown and Transition Year coordinators Sandra Downey, Ann Fitzpatrick, Niamh O'Brien and Jenny Beadle, for your unwavering support during my time there. I know how fortunate I am for the opportunity you gave me.

To Bronagh Starrs for sharing your expertise so generously, and for everything you taught me about adolescent psychotherapy. I couldn't have asked for a better teacher.

To Mary Hilliard for guiding me through some very challenging times in the therapist's chair. Your support was hugely appreciated and much needed.

To Elaine Byrnes for everything you've poured into developing and delivering our TY modules in sexual health over the last number of years, and for all the knowledge and creativity you brought to the creation of our SHARE online course. Many of the examples cited in this book stem from our work together.

To Fergal Brady for always being in my corner.

To Niall Woods and Gemma Cullen for guiding me so well over the past decade.

To Sarah Liddy, in particular, and all the staff at Gill Books for your direction, encouragement and support. Thanks for taking a punt on me again.

And a very special thanks to my wife, Fiona, for lighting up my life on a daily basis as only you can.

Finally, and most importantly of all, to every young person I have met in my work over the past decade. This book is dedicated to you all.